Find Your Roar

A Memoir of Life, Health, and Living with Parkinson's Disease

DEE GIBSON

Published by Market Refined Publishing,
An Imprint of Market Refined Media, LLC
193 Cleo Circle
Ringgold GA 30736
marketrefinedmedia.com

Print ISBN: 979-8-9903602-2-8
Digital ISBN: 979-8-9903602-3-5

LCCN: 2024907245

Cover and Interior Design by Nelly Murariu at PixBeeDesigns.com
Manuscript Edits by Ariel Curry Editorial and Market Refined Media, LLC

Printed in the United States of America

First Edition: April 2024

Dedication

To my one true love, Kathy Gibson, whose life has been a testimony of her love, passion, and patience for me.

And to my three adult children, DeeAnn Hanlon, Andy Gibson, and Denae Green, along with their spouses, and our four incredible grandchildren, Adelyn, Lydia, Gibson, and Marshall, whose love for me has made living with Parkinson's disease less of a challenge.

Thank you all for your unwavering support and encouragement!

CONTENTS

Introduction vii

PART 1: FINDING MY ROAR 1

Chapter 1: My Journey Begins 3

Chapter 2: Mad As Hell 9

Chapter 3: A New Normal 15

Chapter 4: The Quiet Before the Storm 19

Chapter 5: A Year for the Ages 23

Chapter 6: Just Trust Me 27

Chapter 7: My Advocate 31

Chapter 8: Flying Solo 37

Chapter 9: A Peek of What is to Come? 43

Chapter 10: Cheated But Not Defeated 49

Chapter 11: A Rocky Road 59

Chapter 12: Wise Monkeys 67

Chapter 13: In Sickness and Health 73

PART 2: Life in Slow Motion 81

Chapter 14: Kathy's Story: In Her Words 83

Chapter 15: DeeAnn's Story: Superman's Kryptonite 87

Chapter 16: Andy's Story: The Gentle Giant 91

Chapter 17: Denae's Story: The Lifelong Leader 93

PART 3: Is There Purpose in Your Pain? **101**

Chapter 18: Worldview Matters 103

Chapter 19: Loved 109

Epilogue: A Life Worth Living **113**

Acknowledgments 115
Resources 121
Endnotes 125
About the Author 127

INTRODUCTION

It was a crisp fall afternoon just after Thanksgiving in 2019. The sun was peeking in through the sliding glass doors and I was sitting at the kitchen counter "talking" with my son, Andy, about what had become one of my biggest challenges—my speech. The house was silent except for some music playing quietly in the background. There was a scented candle burning in the kitchen with the warm, aromatic smell of vanilla and sugar. It was just the two of us, one of those father and son moments dads always dream of, except that the circumstances that brought us here were less than ideal.

Andy and I were in similar circumstances—well, sort of! Being a leader of a nonprofit in South Carolina, he had just returned home from a time of sabbatical. We were both trying to discern our respective futures. Andy was trying to decide if he was going to stay at his current job, and I was trying to plan for a future that included my recent diagnosis of Parkinson's disease (PD) and figure out how to enjoy my retirement in the meantime. Although I wasn't completely convinced of it, I had been dealing with similar symptoms of PD for over three years. I was still moving pretty well, having just returned from a trip to Washington, D.C., where I had walked and walked and walked some more. But as far as my voice was concerned, it was difficult to speak loud enough to be heard. Andy would lean in whenever I spoke, often putting his ear close to my face to hear what I was saying. Even with the good relationship we had, I was frustrated with him being so close to my face just to hear my voice. I was still holding out hope for a different explanation for my symptoms.

For most people with PD, their voices become softer. In my case, however, I have a hard time getting my words out to begin with. And when I feel stressed or anxious, they often become garbled and almost unintelligible.

As we talked, he shared that he'd been praying for me and believed God would help me "*find my roar.*" Andy felt He would heal my voice, and I prayed he was right. But I also believed God would help me find it in another way. Since that fall afternoon at the kitchen counter with my son, I knew that one day I'd write this book sitting before you now, even though its contents weren't yet fully clear to me in that moment.

This memoir is the record of my journey with Parkinson's disease. Through the depths of my pain, I have had extraordinary experiences with God, my wife Kathy, and my children, which have radically changed the way I live and how I love those around me. In the pages that follow, those suffering with PD, as well as their families and caregivers, will discover that hope can be found even if healing in this life doesn't come. I've learned that a person with this disease can lead a full and meaningful life. In fact, life can be more impactful because chronic pain and suffering keep us more grounded and focused on what is most important in our lives. Despite the circumstances, surrounded by my family's love and being in a right relationship with God reminds me that everything is going to be okay.

Find Your Roar is a book divided into three parts. The first is about my personal journey with Parkinson's. I've heard it said, "*If you've ever met a person with Parkinson's disease, that is exactly what you've done: You have met a* person *with Parkinson's disease.*" You see, what I have learned is that Parkinson's disease, like many other neurological conditions, is very hard to diagnose because it's difficult to discern exactly what is happening with a patient. There are no blood tests or x-rays that can give an exact diagnosis, which can be incredibly frustrating. It is possible many are left wondering, not weeks or months, but often years in trying to determine their exact illness. Not having a firm diagnosis can be more stressful than officially finding out itself.

If this is your diagnosis, I imagine you feel both bewildered and uncertain about your future as well. The unfortunate reality of the situation is it can be extremely difficult to manage your emotions through it. I understand. In part one, I trust that my words and story will help you find hope, peace, and joy in your life.

The second part is about the role and importance of caregivers. I've had the privilege of speaking to a number of those living with PD and those who ultimately provide their care. It's not one person's affliction, but rather a disease that affects an entire family. And as you will see, the closer you are to the person with it, the more your life is changed as well.

The third and final part is about the all-important question of immortality. Is there a purpose in our pain? While this book is primarily for those dealing with PD, I am confident anyone facing a life-altering hardship, suffering, or affliction will find help here. Although this last part of the book is not a deep theological treatise on the question of immortality, it is most definitely a question I have had to wrestle through personally. And I hope anyone who takes the time to read it will find both answers and encouragement. This book is ultimately about hope, healing, and living a life filled with purpose and passion, not in spite of, but because of one's circumstances.

Thank you for going on this journey with me and helping me find my roar. Suffering doesn't have to be the end of the story; rather, it can be the beginning of a new one. My hope and prayer for you is that this book might inspire you to find your *own* roar.

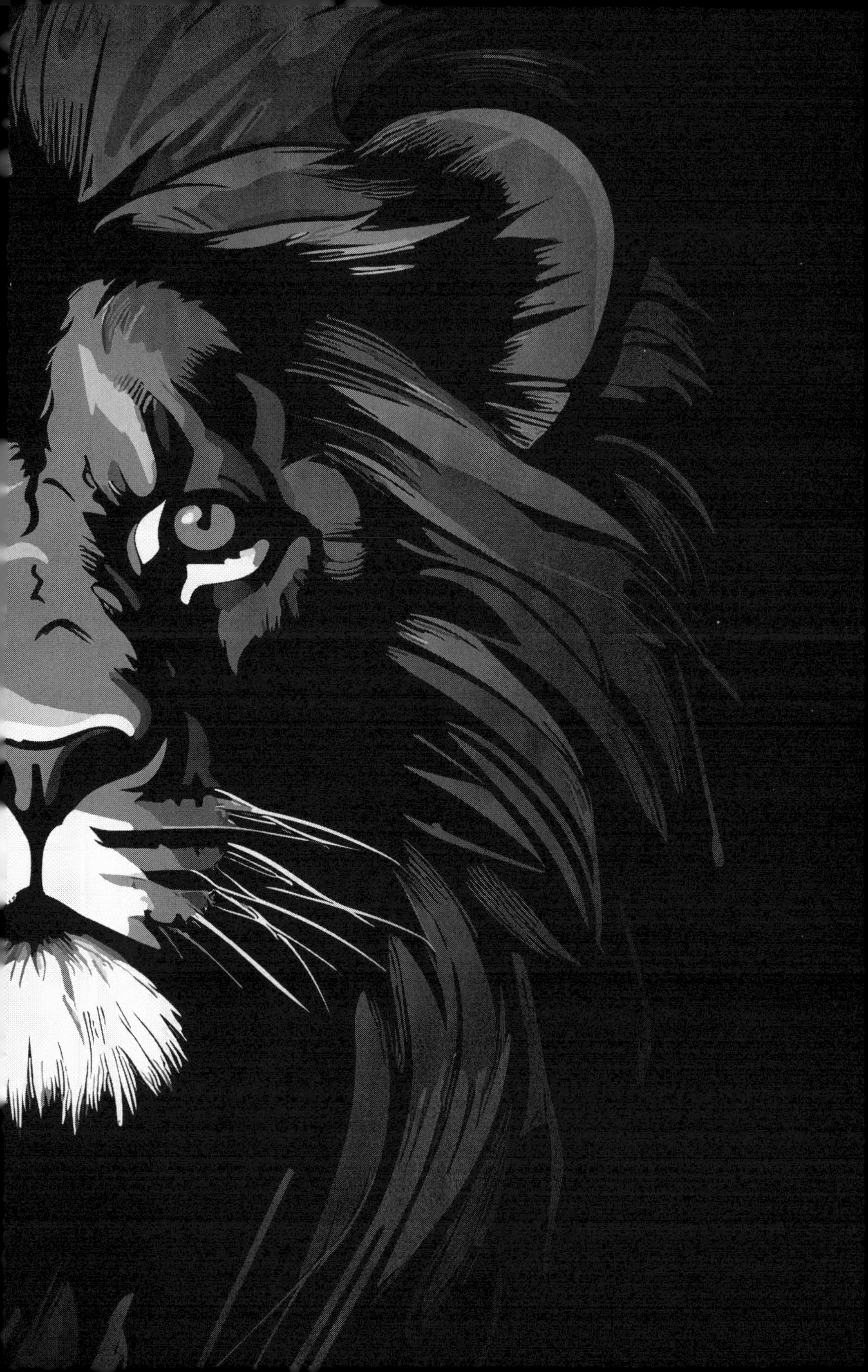

PART 1

Finding My Roar

CHAPTER 1

My Journey Begins

It was early 2015, and I had gone to my primary care doctor for what I thought was a routine office visit. He had known me for years as a big, strong guy. I always prided myself on being physically fit and active, participating in high school sports, running track in college, and playing basketball and lifting weights until my late forties with work colleagues. Even in my early sixties, I retained the athletic build I'd always had. But my doctor had seen some changes. My movement was slower, and my speech had gotten quieter.

"Dee, I want you to go see a neurologist," he told me. "I want to make sure there's nothing going on here."

He knew of patients who could only say a certain number of words in a day, and he didn't want that for me. Some years later, he indicated that because he hadn't seen me very often, he noticed stark changes in my slow movement and gait, what I know today as *bradykinesia*.

I can't say I summarily dismissed his assessment because I went to a follow-up appointment with a neurologist, but I didn't necessarily buy what he was selling, either. In fact, I nearly dismissed the whole notion of having PD after my first visit, primarily because *that* neurologist gives all neurologists a bad name.

As I remember our first visit, he was very cold and distant. He asked me my name and date of birth, then just sat there fiddling around with his ink pen, taking it apart and putting it back together again. He never once looked me in the eye or did any kind of assessment. As I was leaving his office, I considered that a huge waste of my time. I was, and obviously still am, put off by his behavior.

It wasn't until some months later that Kathy, my wife of nearly fifty years, noticed changes in my demeanor as well. We were sitting at the dinner table one evening early in 2016 when she saw I was eating very slowly.

"Dee, are you feeling okay? You remind me of Jim," she said. Jim, my brother-in-law, has waged his own war and battled brilliantly against the same dreaded disease. At this time, I was still an active chief executive officer of a twenty-million-dollar nonprofit called Josiah White's, one of the greatest charitable childcare organizations in the country. It was established in 1850 and created to care for troubled youth in a residential setting. Today, it's one of the largest childcare institutions in Indiana with a vast array of services, including residential treatment, therapeutic foster care, and home-based services for teens and their families. On top of my work there, I was still jogging (albeit ever so slowly), swimming laps, and weightlifting.

As time progressed, I noticed changes in my ability to swim laps. My arm motion was not as smooth or flexible as it had been earlier. Until a few years ago, our family would often go out in the boat at the lake to swim and bathe during the summers. We would take shampoo and lather up, and then jump into the lake for our daily bath. I am now, however, like a beached whale because I must watch from the boat. I can no longer swim well enough to stay afloat or get in and out of the boat with ease.

I have a very good friend, Jim, who, for a couple of years, worked in a senior living community with a swimming pool. After Jim retired from the Federal Motor Carrier Safety Administration, he was a lifeguard at the pool and assisted elderly people, a number of whom had PD. He told me he would often have to put ankle weights on clients so they wouldn't lose their balance and end up upside down in the pool. I hate to say it, but for a season in my life, I dismissed Jim's comments because I felt what he was saying didn't apply to me. Now, however, it makes perfect sense. As my Parkinson's has progressed over the last six years, what originally was slow movement became muscle rigidity and is now postural instability.

A second early warning sign was my quiet voice, although it was still much louder and more understandable at the time than it is today. Other people had commented on my tone and volume as well, but I shrugged it off as possible nerve damage from a throat surgery some years prior.

Yet another early sign was my handwriting, but then again, I've always had terrible writing skills, even from a young age. I was a southpaw (left-handed), which meant I constantly wrote over the top of words I'd just written. My handwriting was so poor I often quipped that I wrote like a third grader. Truth be told, my grandson, who *is* a third grader, has great penmanship. But today, my handwriting is so poor that I avoid writing as much as I possibly can. As an adult, however, there are times when writing my name, address, phone number, and email address are unavoidable. This has turned into one of my biggest embarrassments because I write so small it's utterly unintelligible. Even with some occupational therapy, nothing has proven helpful to date. Thank goodness I can still type reasonably well, which has been a godsend when it comes to my communication skills!

And finally, a fourth early warning sign was a "frozen shoulder" which can be very painful. Going back close to fifteen years, I had the first of two secondary shoulder impingements. Simple daily tasks can become almost impossible to do—things like putting on a belt or coat or tucking in your shirt. But I can tell you as painful as these things are, the treatment modalities are worse and downright barbaric.

I believed at times that my physical therapist was a sadist. There are fibers that grow together and restrict your movement, much like a rubber band that is pulled tight all the time. They impede your arm's ability to move freely in the joint. My physical therapist's job was to break these rubber band-like structures in my arm to allow for freedom of movement. The problem wasn't so much the therapist as it was the home treatments he assigned, which involved things like broomsticks and Kathy using her leverage to manipulate my arm in ways it simply didn't want to go. Although she hated putting me through the pain, we had some fun with the whole "broom" thing, specifically when I accused her of being the "wicked witch of the west." Actually, Kathy would be an excellent physical therapist. She liked to say, "I know this is going to hurt, but do it anyway!"

The formal definition of a frozen shoulder is when the humeral head isn't centered within the shoulder joint, causing impingement when the arm is moved. Common causes include specific upper body exercises, poor posture, or muscle imbalances such as rotator cuff weakness. The working theory is that this condition is due to a change in the arm swing of people with PD. The good news is that if you are willing to go through the pain of rehabilitation, my experience has been that you can recover from a frozen shoulder, even with a Parkinson's diagnosis.

Because of Kathy's concerns, I went to see another neurologist at the Indiana University Medical Center, but I still wasn't convinced. They explained the difficulty in diagnosing PD, primarily because the symptoms are so varied and elusive. He was not prepared to give a conclusive finding, especially given that my symptoms were so mild then. He did, however, suggest I consider Rock Steady Boxing. It's a nationally recognized program in Indianapolis, and it's known to benefit those with Parkinson's.

Kathy and I stopped by the gym on our way home. One of the original founders was a lady who showed me around, and she proudly proclaimed they were known as "the badasses of PD." The Rock Steady Boxing program has four different levels; the lowest level is designed for those with only mild symptoms. I was impressed with the entire program. They had good facilities with all the equipment needed to teach boxing, but most of all, they had the right attitude towards the disease. I even joined another location closer to my home and attended classes regularly for the next year until my thyroid cancer surgery. I went weekly to the Level One class, where we did all kinds of boxing drills which I had never done before, but I really enjoyed the training. I used the heavy bag and beat the snot out of it. Fortunately, for everyone involved, there was no live contact between clients.

Although I don't remember much about those early months in the class, I can recall with clarity the founder's comment about being a badass. I felt like one and didn't realize how much I needed it. In fact, that comment means more to me today, given the progression of the disease I've seen in my own life. Still, throughout 2016, I struggled to accept the reality of the disease, in part because my symptoms were so mild and because the neurologist at the IU Medical Center hesitated to give me a firm diagnosis. Soon, however, I wouldn't be able to ignore the signs any longer.

CHAPTER 2

Mad As Hell

It was a cold, wintery night on the twenty-eighth of February 2017. It was three o'clock in the morning, and I was lying in a hospital bed recovering from the second of two surgeries to remove my thyroid. I felt unsettled in my spirit—not so much afraid, but anxious! Emotional! Worried! I wasn't even certain about what.

I suspect part of my anxiety was a lack of sleep. The night before the surgery, I showered with a special soap to prevent infection, which only added to my anxiety. It was the moment I realized this was not a standard routine procedure. And then I had to be at the hospital before dawn.

After surgery, and throughout the day and night, the nursing staff came into my room checking my vitals and all the tubes attached to my body. I had been pricked and probed in every way imaginable and felt like a proverbial pin cushion. But hey, at least I knew the ropes. Two weeks earlier, I'd had the exact same surgery. The first was to remove just half of my thyroid, in hopes the cancer would be contained in the nodule itself and a full thyroid removal wouldn't be necessary. But it was.

I HAVE THYROID CANCER! There is something very sobering about hearing the words, "You have cancer," that causes a person to stop and evaluate their life. This was a gut check moment . . . when I realized I was getting older and as the Good Book says:

> *"You've limited our life span to a mere seventy years, yet some you give grace to live still longer. But even the best of years are marred by tears and toils and in the end are nothing more than a gravestone in a graveyard! We're gone so quickly, so swiftly; we pass away and simply disappear."* (Psalm 90:10 TPT)

Up to this point in my life, I had felt pretty good. Sure, I'd had some health concerns, including the suspected PD a year earlier, but overall, it had not yet seriously affected my life. But now, with my thyroid removed because of cancer, I was taking inventory. I came to understand all too well the truth of this verse. My days are numbered.

I've never considered myself a poet but had limited exposure to it through some of our students at Josiah White's. They were young, teenage men from troubled backgrounds, and they wrote incredible poetry under the guidance of house parents who had worked with a professor at Manchester University. Reading their words, I determined that when I retired, I would write some poetry too. Little did I realize these first two would take on such a significant role in my life. The following poem, titled "Mad as Hell," was written over the two weeks following my first surgery—starting at three o'clock in the morning on that lonely, hospital bed in the Indiana University Medical Center.

POEM ONE

"Mad as Hell"

They say sometimes you win some
And sometimes you lose some.
And right now, I'm mad as Hell.

I had my life all planned out neat, tidy, and with a bow.
But life has dealt me a really big blow.
And right now, I'm mad as Hell.

When an incurable disease enters your life
And all the plans you had no longer likely to survive
With all of life's hopes, dreams, and pleasures now in doubt
And when purpose, value, and worth seem so elusive
I wonder what will come of me.
With each passing day, I'm reminded
I'm not the man I used to be.
And right now, I'm mad as Hell.

Coming to terms with a future where
Intimate walks, leisurely bike rides, and making love
With *My One and Only* will no longer be,
And my lover will become my caregiver.
And right now, I'm mad as Hell.

Like a thief in the night
Being robbed of life's most treasured possessions,
Knowing the day will come when time and esteem from my
Children will wane and I'll be left behind no longer the
Strong leader of our family, only
The one who will require care and accommodation.
And right now, I'm mad as Hell.

As the hourglass of my life runs out
And my worth in the eyes of others now in doubt,
From CEO leading the way to a CEO leading from behind
All because this dreaded disease is taking my ability to
Write, speak, and set the pace.
And right now, I'm mad as Hell.

They say sometimes you win some,
Sometimes you lose some.
And right now, I'm losing bad.

In the weeks following my second surgery, I wrote part two, with tubes hanging out of my throat to drain excess blood from the incision. This time of significant pain and discomfort was when I began to grapple with the reality of my new life.

The second half of this poem was inspired by a song entitled, "Even If", by the Christian group Mercy Me, which had been released a short time prior. I heard the lead singer explain the backstory for the lyrics and it spoke to me in a way that drove me to tears. His son had been diagnosed with a form of autism that plagued their family for years. And even though many have prayed for his deliverance, as of the writing of this book, the son has not been healed. This song took on even greater significance for me after hearing about this man's fatherly love and that *even if* God chose not to heal him, he trusted for His goodness and grace. I resolved to find my own way to praise Him by writing a second poem, *even if* I wasn't healed.

I had given up trying to control everything at Josiah White's some years earlier. It was simply too big and too complex. I had given up trying to be in control of my finances; after all, it all belongs to the Big Man upstairs anyway! And now perhaps, for the very first time, I was coming to terms with the fact that I don't have control over my health either. Regardless of how hard I tried, I now realized my health was in God's hands too.

POEM TWO

In Christ Alone

With all these doubts, fears,
And seemingly unattainable dreams
I realize my life is not my own.
I'm a steward of this body—this life, not the owner.
It is not my will, but His will be done.
My hope is in Christ alone!
I know God is able, I know He can
Put all the pieces back together again.
Like Job of the Bible, I cannot curse God.
My hope is in Christ alone.

I know God is able, I know He can
Like Meshach, Shadrach, and Abednego
Be guided through the flames to safety again.
I cannot be angry.
My hope is in Christ alone.

I know God is able, I know He can
Remove all this pain and doubt.
But even if He doesn't,
Help me to remember
My hope is in Christ alone.
And when my days have come to an end
Help me to sing loud and clear
It is well—it is well with my soul.

CHAPTER 3

A New Normal

After being released from the surgeon's care, my life returned to more of a normal pace and routine. He told me from the beginning of my diagnosis that this cancer was very treatable, and the chance of me dying from it were slight. I believed him, and once again, I was consumed by my duties of being a CEO.

Because I had planned on retiring at the end of 2017, my final ten months at Josiah White's were different from previous years. Much of my time was spent with the succession planning committee of the board and celebrating with co-workers and friends while closing out a forty-year career.

In the last twenty years, I had worked very closely with the board of directors. On one particular occasion, I had a breakfast meeting with a long-term member. We were sitting in a quaint, little restaurant called The Fried Egg, discussing my retirement when I mustered up the courage to discuss my PD diagnosis with her.

"I think I have Parkinson's disease," I finally blurted out. Tears welled up in her eyes in what I initially thought was pity but turned out to be relief. Some board members had expressed concern to her and wondered if there wasn't something more seriously wrong, perhaps even a terminal illness I had not shared with them, because they had not yet decided who would be replacing me. Up until this point, I had dodged the whole discussion with the board (and everyone else for that matter), blaming all my more visible symptoms on cancer. It was obvious to those who knew me very well that there were things

I was trying to conceal. Probably the most obvious difference was in my voice. Whether in board meetings or at social events, I simply didn't have the strength in my vocal cords to project my voice and produce the same confidence I had prior to the onset of PD. And when walking with them, I had trouble keeping up. Most people knew something happened physically, but because I was struggling with coming to terms with it myself, I ignored and side-stepped any conversation about my health with anyone other than my closest family. I was in denial.

Fortunately for me, my youngest and very talented daughter, Denae, was the director of communications at Josiah White's. And Kathy, my incredible wife and administrative assistant during my entire tenure as CEO, ran interference for me. For virtually any public event I attended, one or both were at my side helping me communicate and share the message of the impact of Josiah White's. Without them, I doubt I would have made it!

Denae helped prepare my public remarks whenever I spoke and was always close by me. Kathy often became my interpreter when we met with donors. Near the end of my time there, I began sharing my health issues with selected donors and colleagues, all the while still holding out hope that Parkinson's was not the correct and final diagnosis. I didn't want to admit I had this life-altering disease. All of the donors, however, were very gracious, and because I had close relationships with them, they loved and accepted me with grace.

As my time as CEO wound down, I felt it couldn't come quickly enough. I was tired of talking to people, both trying to hide my PD from some and trying to share what I thought was going on with others. And then, on December 31, 2017, the big day arrived, and without any fanfare or even a big New Year's Eve party to attend, I was retired!

I invested virtually all my adult life into Josiah White's, making it hard to put into words what I felt on that particular evening. It was a mixture of excitement about what our new future might be as well as a sense of anxiety about the unknown, particularly surrounding my health. But primarily, there was a relief knowing I was no longer responsible for this incredible institution. It was time to start the next chapter of our lives. And we did!

Being at Josiah White's organization for forty years was an incredible blessing. One of the biggest perks of the job was campus housing. I had enjoyed living in the director's home for twenty years, which was not only a huge blessing but also a big curse because we had to move all the stuff we had naturally accumulated over the years. We raised all three of our now-adult children in that home. And I recognized it as a sign the staff knew I wasn't doing well when they wouldn't let me help move our furniture and personal belongings. Even the students gently ushered me off to the side, insisting this was what they were getting paid to do. But everyone there that day knew why I was sitting this one out.

For the next eight months, Kathy and I lived at our condo on Lake Webster while our new home was being built in Sweetser, Indiana. We chose to build a new home rather than buy an existing home, in large part because down deep in the pit of my stomach, I knew this proverbial sea monster lurking just below the surface of the water would one day come roaring up to take away my mobility and whatever else I was willing to concede.

We were able to build a home with zero transition, which simply means we have a home with no steps, including no steps from our garage into our home. We also made the doorways larger. Most standard doors are two feet, eight inches" by six feet, eight inches, but we actually made ours a full thirty-six inches wide, allowing for wheelchair accessibility throughout the home. And finally, we installed bars along our bathroom and shower walls. These additions were made at some additional cost but have already proven to be very helpful to me, as well as a number of our family and friends.

I am now five years in our new home, and I have yet to need a wheelchair. But with my walking as unpredictable as it is, I realize I'm one fall away from needing one. This was just one sign of how I was slowly coming to understand and accept the life ahead of me.

CHAPTER 4

The Quiet Before the Storm

We moved into our new home at the end of July 2018. In August, I started my next grand adventure, which was becoming a Colson Fellow.

The Colson Fellowship program is a rigorous ten-month deep dive into interpreting our ever-changing culture through the lens of an unchanging Christian worldview. Starting in August 2018 to May 2019, I committed roughly twenty hours a week to reading scripture and numerous books on relevant topics affecting our culture. I considered applying to become a Colson Fellow for some time and knew I needed something productive to do with my time after retirement. This was exactly what I needed. The program was challenging and yet very rewarding.

But first, I had to take care of another impending health concern.

Way back as a junior in high school, I was injured in a football game. It's amazing to me I can still remember the team we were playing, the time of the game, and even the play itself. At any rate, for many years, I walked around feeling a bit like Captain Hook with a peg leg. So, in January 2019, after having consulted with my doctors, I decided to have a full knee replacement on the right side. I had always heard this was a painful surgery, and the therapy required afterward was extremely painful too. And they were right. But I can tell you with certainty it was even more difficult for Kathy because of the timing and the care required afterward.

My surgery was scheduled for bright and early on January 30, 2019. Kathy and I decided to make the ninety-minute trip to the hospital the night before so, as my grandsons would say, *we wouldn't have to get up at the butt crack of dawn*. I remember this clearly because the outside temperature was a frigid twenty-two degrees below zero. The only colder days ever recorded in Indiana's books were the next two days. My ever-faithful wife, Kathy, traversed the frigid temperatures and snow-covered highways just to be at my side. Now that is love!

After two nights in the hospital, we made the trek back home. Once there, though, I was very lethargic. I couldn't keep my eyes open and literally could not put one foot in front of the other. I have often joked that I felt like a drunken sailor, although, to be honest, I don't really know how it feels to be a drunken sailor! Fortunately, Denae lived close by and came over to help me get out of the car and into the house. After a brief trip to the bathroom, I wasn't able to make the transition from there to my bed. While I wasn't able to move, I did have enough mental capacity to suggest they could get me from the bathroom to the bed with the help of my office chair. There is much about that day of coming home from the hospital I do not remember, however, I do recall both Kathy and Denae being at least mildly impressed that I had enough mental faculties to make the chair a workable option to haul my not-so-tiny behind from one room to the next.

After a few frantic phone calls, Kathy discovered they had changed my medication the morning we left the hospital, and I was having a reaction to the new pain medication. But once this was corrected, I began to feel better with each passing day. I'm not sure how my PD factored into my reaction to the medication, but I can say with confidence I don't recall ever having problems with any medications prescribed to me prior to my Parkinson's medication regimen.

My commissioning as a Colson Fellow was at the end of May in Washington, D.C., and I was on a mission to make that trip without crutches or other medical assistance. After much physical therapy following the surgery, I was able to attend, along with Kathy, my daughter DeeAnn, and my granddaughter Adylen. I had just come through a full knee replacement four months prior to my commissioning, and I successfully walked to the podium to receive my certificate. That was a big deal to me! I had worked really hard in the program, and it set the stage for me to actually put pen to paper and write this book.

In the last quarter of the program, every Colson Fellow was asked to write a personal mission statement and three-year ministry plan. And although it took me a while longer to write my personal mission statement and put my plan into action, I was able to finally compile it . . . and what you are reading today is a big part of my plan. What follows is my Mission and Vision Statement:

> *My mission is to be a Godly example to all in my sphere of influence, but especially to men and those struggling with disabilities. My vision is to minister to men of all ages (4-94) so they may become Godly men and pass their faith on to future generations. And because God has allowed me to have PD, I would like to be a source of encouragement to those who are fellow laborers who are fighting this fight along with me. I hope to start a blog and/or write a book detailing my challenges with PD.*

Another milestone for me on this trip was being able to walk with DeeAnn and Adelyn to all the main sites and even able to take a tour of the White House without using any crutches or assistance devices.

I realize today just how fortunate I was to be able to go to Washington, D.C. Although I knew I had this diagnosis looming in the background of my mind, given that I had come through the surgery so well and was able to navigate all the walking as well as I did, I wondered again if I actually had PD, or if my problems were perhaps more skeletal in nature.

A few months later, the official diagnosis came—I had Parkinson's disease. Seeing the label there on paper—now an undeniable fact—was quite a jolt to my heart and mind. To be completely honest, I'm not sure why I earned this less-than-honorable distinction of having PD because in my mind, nothing had changed. Both my symptoms and level of functioning were the same. And yet here I sat with an official diagnosis. I have since learned the uncertainty of *do I, or don't I* officially have this dreaded disease is the case for about half of all Parkinson's patients. Little did I know these final months of 2019 would be the last bit of normalcy I would have until the writing of this book.

CHAPTER 5

A Year for the Ages

It was not your typical Indiana January 6 by anyone's standard. In fact, by Indiana weather standards, it was almost balmy. My oldest grandson, who was five at the time, conned me to go outside with him to play some catch with the football in the yard.

It all happened so fast. One minute, I was upright doing the Super Bowl shuffle, and the next minute I was laying in the middle of our driveway, completely and totally embarrassed, not because I had fallen, but because my five-year-old grandson had just scored on me. What started out as a game of catch quickly turned into him running toward an imaginary goal and me moving laterally to stop him from scoring an imaginary touchdown. I remember feeling stiff and not flexible like I did prior to my days with Parkinson's. But even so, I was not going to let my grandson get the best of me . . . at least that was the plan! How is it that a sixty-five-year-old former football player can't even keep up with his five-year-old grandson? It's easy; this man has PD. And as much as I tried to ignore that reality, it snuck up and bit me in the ass (*figuratively speaking*, of course)!

When I fell that dreadful day, I fell hard. My left hip hurt like crazy, but I had no idea the events of that morning would still be impacting me to this day. I remember thinking, "Wow! This really hurts and I'm going to have a heck of a bruise." All the while my grandson, Gibson, was doing his own version of a touchdown celebration. We were both unaware of what would transpire over the next several months. I sat on the driveway in a bit of a daze, assessing the damage and dealing with the embarrassment of my neighbors seeing me fall. But thankfully, I was able to get up of my own accord.

Over the next three days, I suffered, not just physically but also mentally, for two reasons. I had been beaten in a game of pick-up football by my grandson, and I feared something was seriously wrong with my hip because it wasn't getting any better. After three days, I went to my family doctor for some x-rays, and to my unexpected relief, they said they didn't see any fractures or breaks. So, I tried to be a tough guy and gut out all the pain I was feeling in my hip. I imagined myself like Bruce Willis in the 1988 Christmas movie *Die Hard*, where he was shot at and beaten up, but was still able to run miles at a time to avoid capture and shoot the next bad guy every time!

What I didn't realize was that because I was in so much pain and stopped moving normally in those three weeks, my muscles were atrophying. They were getting weaker and weaker by the day to the point that even now, two years later, I'm still trying to regain the muscle mass lost during this time.

A month later, I was still living in pain. We had just gone to bed and the unthinkable happened. I turned over and experienced the most excruciating pain tear through my body, like I was being mauled by a grizzly bear. My hip had displaced, meaning the femur broke off at the neck, just below the ball going into my hip socket. I instantly knew this was something serious and was not going to improve anytime soon. But I had another more immediate problem to deal with before anyone else could be called in for reinforcements.

You see, for most of my married life, I slept in the buff—butt naked and not a stitch of clothing. So picture this—well, okay, maybe *don't* picture this—but try to understand my dilemma. I was lying in bed with the most unbearable pain one can imagine. And I needed to get underwear on so I could call an ambulance and make sure my daughter wouldn't have to live with the mental picture of seeing her dad in all his glory! With a lot of help from Kathy, who was as concerned as I was about the prospect of everyone seeing me in my birthday suit, I was able to get through the agony of finally slipping on a pair of my underwear. We waited for what seemed like eternity for the ambulance and my daughter to arrive, but it was actually just under fifteen minutes.

In between my cries of pain, we discussed how the ambulance should make its grand entrance into our home and agreed it shouldn't be with sirens blaring at 11:30 p.m. Somehow, that just didn't seem fitting to us. After all, it wasn't like this was a true emergency or anything! Once the paramedics arrived, I mistakenly thought the worst was over, certain they would give me some strong drugs to put me in ignorant bliss. Boy, was I wrong! They informed me that they were going to roll me on my side to put a blanket under my thankfully now covered derrière, and I needed to be prepared for it to hurt. Once I was finally situated, they carted me outside to my awaiting chariot, which rode more like a chuckwagon to the hospital. It didn't help that I was shivering, partly because I wasn't sure what to make of my newfound predicament but also because it was freezing cold.

Once at the hospital, they got medication flowing through my veins, and I believe it was morphine. Whatever it was, it did the trick, and I felt much better, at least for the moment. My incredibly faithful wife stuck by my bedside surely thinking, "Here we go again!" And *here we go again* was exactly right.

Less than thirty-six hours after my femur broke, I was moved to a trauma surgeon at an Indianapolis hospital to have emergency hip replacement surgery. It had been one year within a matter of ten days that she nursed me through my knee replacement, and now this! When Kathy uttered those marriage vows at that small Quaker church, just outside Marion, Indiana, promising to stick with me in sickness and in health, I can't imagine she had any idea our life would be like this.

I was beginning to understand the meaning of those vows in a way I had never considered before! This time, I was in the hospital for two weeks. If there was any good news throughout this whole ordeal, it wasn't much. But at least COVID-19 had not hit the hospital yet.

Neither one of us realized this was just the warmup act of what was to come ten months later. From my surgery in February through mid-December 2020, my life was fairly normal for a Parkinson's patient. My weekdays were spent in physical and speech therapy, and my focus was on regaining the ability to walk normally. During that ten-month period, I went to three different physical therapists, each with their own set of strengths. But I have learned the importance of finding someone who has the skills, experience, and temperament to work with Parkinson's patients, starting with a basic understanding of what they may be experiencing physically. Life in the "recovery lane" can be a bit more complicated because they do not have the flexibility and balance of more normal patients. A good PT should understand what kind of exercises are best suited for PD patients. And probably most important to me is having a therapist with the patience to work with someone who cannot accomplish tasks with the same level of proficiency as a person without this disease.

I mentioned to Kathy that I felt I had been progressing nicely to the point of once again feeling almost normal. While I still had a bit of a limp, I was able to ambulate around without the use of crutches, canes, or walkers. That is, until that fateful day one week before Christmas in 2020.

CHAPTER 6

Just Trust Me

The date that will live on in infamy for the rest of our lives is December 17, 2020. Kathy and I were on our way home from her eye doctor appointment in Marion. I had been to the YMCA earlier that week and was feeling great. The appointment ran late into the afternoon because the doctor diagnosed her with a detached retina. She had surgery scheduled for the next day in Indianapolis, so we headed home to try for a good night's sleep.

It was dark outside, just a few minutes after 6:00 p.m. Snow had been falling, and Kathy was in the passenger seat with her eyes closed. As we were driving home on a lightly traveled road about four miles from our home, a pick-up truck ran a stop sign and hit us on my side, going about fifty-five miles per hour. The impact was immediate, swift, and disorienting—much like a football player who gets blindsided in pursuit of an opposing team's running back. The only memory I have of the moments preceding the truck slamming into us is a quick glimpse of its headlights about a half-mile up the road. But from that moment on, the truck was in my blind spot. The next thing I recall is the impact.

Immediately, I knew what had happened. The airbags exploded, spewing white powder all over us. Kathy and I both had big bottles of water in the car, and when mixed with the powder, we both looked a little like Casper the friendly ghost. The car had just stopped sliding through the barren cornfield when I heard Kathy say, "What just happened?" To the best of my ability, I told her what she already knew. We had been in an accident. Even at this moment, my speech was not very strong. Darn PD!

Our car had barely stopped moving when I heard a voice coming from outside the car saying, "Are you guys okay?"

"Don't get out of the car," he said. "There are power lines down. Help is on the way." And sure enough, within a minute or two, there were more people asking if I was okay. Meanwhile, back inside the car, Kathy was checking to see if I could move my fingers and toes, and I responded affirmatively. All the while, I was fumbling around to find my phone. It was like trying to find a needle in a haystack, but once I found it, I called Denae. It was a phone call no one ever wants to get, but I figured it was best coming from me rather than from a police officer.

One of the things I have learned to really appreciate about Denae is her ability to navigate through a crisis. While at Josiah White's, we had our share of them, and she had proven to be capable and calm in any situation that arose.

When I shared with her that we were in an accident, she promptly asked me if we were okay. I told her I thought so but we were pretty shaken up. She asked where the accident was and if 911 had been called, and I said yes. She then indicated she would meet us at the hospital. Within minutes, I was approached by a man and woman who identified themselves as from the fire department. Thankfully, they took over the entire situation and were both very reassuring as well as capable in assessing our needs. Because the truck hit me square on my driver's side door, the first order of business was getting my car door open. The "Jaws of Life" have new meaning now that I have seen them in action. Once the door was cut away, they asked if I thought I could walk because we ended up out in the field and it would be difficult to get the stretcher out to the car. My adrenaline must have been off the charts because I remember walking a hundred yards through a semi-frozen plowed field from my car to the ambulance with a neck brace on and thinking I had not only escaped with my life, but also my health.

Kathy's circumstances were much the same, but she indicated later the feeling of her back being displaced. She too was able to walk out of the field where we were then separated into two different ambulances with the assurance of being back together at the hospital. I think everyone we encountered instinctively knew that we were two-peas-in-a-pod. For a long time, Kathy and I have had this little thing we say to each other: "We go together like peanut butter and jelly, salt and pepper, cookies and milk." You get the picture.

Once at the hospital, doctors did all kinds of tests and exams on me and Kathy. We were in the emergency room with only a curtain separating us. Throughout the entire ordeal, Denae responded with incredible poise and calm. She was our go-between, relaying messages back and forth and making sure each of our respective doctors and nurses knew that I had Parkinson's disease and that Kathy had a detached retina.

After they looked me over from head to toe, inside and out, I was starting to feel all the pain from my injuries. What I did not realize was the extent of them, that is until one of the doctors told me they thought I had some internal bleeding in and around my heart that could be life-threatening, so they were sending me to Lutheran Hospital in Fort Wayne. Needless to say, this was somewhat of a jolt because I didn't feel like I was going to die. In fact, over the next several hours, I wondered more than once if this was what it felt like to be on my deathbed. They initially planned to life flight me by helicopter but quickly changed their minds and decided to send me by ambulance instead. With the high winds, they didn't feel it was safe to fly. I was disappointed because I'd never flown in a helicopter and was looking forward to it. *Hey, if I was going to die, I figured I might as well go out doing something exciting!* Rather than a twenty-minute ride by helicopter, I was sentenced to a bumpy, hour-plus ride by ambulance.

I was really feeling the pain of my serious injuries, and they gave me medication to make the trip a bit easier. But most importantly, I had a chance to see Kathy before I left. She was lying on one stretcher, and I was on the other. We held hands and whispered a prayer for one another before I was whisked away to the ambulance.

I always knew how important my relationship was with my family, but on this particular night, I realized just how important and how deep my love was for Kathy and my kids. Having that simple, little prayer and moment together before I left was so very important to me. It was that small reassurance that said, “We are all going to get through this and be together again.”

Although I have no recollection of what we talked about, I remember making small talk with the EMT, just to pass the time. Other than it being a very bumpy ride, all the small talk made us miss the exit to the hospital not once, but twice. So here I am being transported by ambulance to a facility roughly an hour away because I have life-threatening injuries, and the driver gets distracted and passes the entrance! Thankfully, I was still in shock and didn’t fully comprehend my brush with mortality because if I had, I would have been freaking out.

There have been a handful of times in my life where I knew God had an angel watching over me. I believe this to be one of those times. When I whispered those short little prayers, it seems He answered them in ways I will only see when I get to heaven. For the second time in less than six hours, I felt God assured me that everyone was going to be okay.

CHAPTER 7

My Advocate

I arrived safely at Lutheran Hospital, and after further testing and assessment by the trauma team, they determined there was no bleeding around my heart. It was just a big bruise on my chest where I had a fractured sternum, in addition to a broken left clavicle, three fractured vertebrae, and several fractured ribs. Once I realized I wasn't going to die, my focus returned to Kathy. She was also in intensive care, but now desperately needed surgery on her eye.

Unbeknownst to me, Kathy, Denae, and my oldest daughter DeeAnn, a nurse living in Tallahassee, FL, all had been working behind the scenes to figure out what to do next. As a result, Kathy was released from intensive care the following morning to go to her eye surgery and then home to recuperate. I later learned this was the one and only time during the height of COVID that our kids had to divide and conquer our continued care. Denae was responsible for Kathy, Andy was responsible for me, and DeeAnn would provide her expertise from Tallahassee until she could get a flight to Indiana.

Kathy and the kids determined that after my release from the hospital, I would need to go to a rehab center. I reluctantly agreed for Kathy's sake, because I knew she also needed some serious healing before she could even consider helping me. I required extensive help to shower and go to the bathroom, let alone walk. The result was a two-week stay at a rehab in Fort Wayne. The kids called multiple rehab facilities only to be told that once I was admitted, because of

COVID-19 restrictions, I would not be able to have any visitors. They found one facility in Fort Wayne that had a different policy. At this facility, I was allowed just one visitor who could come and go as they pleased for the next two weeks. Since Andy had drawn the short end of the stick and been assigned to me, it was boys' time for the next two weeks.

That is time I hope to never repeat again, and not because of Andy—he was a lifeline for me. But it was the first time in more than forty-five years I had been away from Kathy for that long. On top of that, I was admitted to the rehab facility on the twenty-second of December, which meant I would be away from Kathy and the kids on Christmas, New Year's Eve, and Kathy's birthday in early January. Since we married, we had never been apart on all these big family days.

My first few days at the rehab facility were the worst. The little trip across town from the hospital to the rehab facility was refreshing, but very cold. While it was nice being outside for a bit, I had to go pee pretty badly and decided to wait to get to my new "pad" before emptying my ever-bloating bladder. When I initially asked the nurse about going to the bathroom, she insisted I go while lying flat on my back, which I knew wouldn't to happen. Eventually, the nurse agreed to let me go if she could stand beside the bed to make sure I didn't fall. I told her I had a bad case of "stage fright" and that wasn't going to happen either. She wasn't going to give me a break, though, so I waited and waited and waited some more until I finally had a "come to Jesus" meeting with the in-charge nurse who finally agreed to let me stand beside my bed by myself, as long as I promised not to fall. I promised, and let it rip! I completely filled one plastic portable urinal to the brim.

This was the first of a few run-ins with the nurses. I remember thinking this was going to be a couple of long weeks if this was the way it was going to be.

One of the big selling points of going to a rehab facility was that I could get all the intensive therapy needed. I was supposed to have a minimum of three hours of therapy every day (one hour each of physical, occupational, and speech), but because it was the twenty-second of December when I arrived, everybody and their brother was off for at least four days. I grew angrier by the hour as I contemplated my predicament. There was no way I was going to stay there through the holidays if I wasn't even going to be getting therapy. So, instead, I lay in the hospital bed for the first three days, planning my escape.

But it was Andy to the rescue! Fortunately, he has excellent communication skills, and I needed him to use them. After I briefed him on my concerns and frustrations, he asked for a meeting with the hospital personnel involved in my care. The meeting occurred the day after Christmas and obviously, for me, the day could not come soon enough. To say I was impressed with Andy and the rehab facility doesn't do justice for the meeting that transpired that day. I'm not sure how Andy got everyone there, but the afternoon of the meeting, the room was full of people, including two doctors, the entire team of physical, occupational, and speech therapists, the nursing staff, and even a rehab facility administrator.

"You have the opportunity to change my dad's life," he told them. He said that he felt the system was getting in the way of my care, and the communication between staff was poor. He shared a few examples of how the staff let me down in my care. Having had some time to reflect on the events of those terribly stressful and dark days, I have come away with three key takeaways.

First is the importance of having a healthcare advocate. I realized that day I was not capable of advocating for myself. I've always appreciated Steven Covey's book, *The Seven Habits of Highly Effective People*. His first habit is to begin with the end in mind. And I simply was in no way capable of being able to consider what I needed long-term. I was still reeling from the accident and all that had transpired up to that point. I needed help, and thankfully, I had my kids there.

Second, Andy, along with some help from my other two kids, came up with a list of key questions I think would be great for anyone who is going into any type of extended care, be it intensive rehab, assisted living, or even skilled care. Below is a sample of the kinds of questions I found helpful:

1. **Do I have an advocate for my care?** I can't overstate the importance of having someone in your corner, ready to be your advocate when you are not capable of representing yourself.
2. **Who is in charge of my care?** What physician is ultimately responsible? Where does the buck stop? I think it's incredibly important that an individual be responsible. While I appreciate the importance of teams, from the perspective of the one receiving care, there needs to be one person who can make final decisions.
3. **Who will I be working with?** In my case, I had five different physical therapists during my first five days of care, which I understand and appreciate, as it was over the Christmas holidays, but it is important that a person be provided with continuity of care. I would suggest having introductions at an original team meeting, much like I had five days into my care, only more proactively done.
4. **When will I be discharged from care?** This is obviously an important question for the one receiving care. But beyond having a clear sense of when I would be released, it also drove a lot of other questions as well. For example, how much physical, speech, and occupational therapy would I be receiving, and who would be responsible for coordinating my care after I was discharged from an acute rehab facility?
5. The last big question for any acute care staff is this: **What would they say the prognosis is, both the best- and worst-case scenarios?** We all understand the acute care facility walks a tightrope balancing act between continuing to demonstrate the need for continued care and showing adequate progress to provide some light at the end of the tunnel to the insurance company.

Once the meeting had concluded, the level of care I received almost immediately improved dramatically. The hospital administrator even gave permission for Kathy to have extended opportunities to visit me during the height of the COVID-19 lockdown. She came to see me on Christmas day and her birthday, even though I'm sure she didn't feel well herself because she was still recovering from her eye surgery and a host of injuries from the accident. Just to see her smiling face meant the world to me. I was reminded of the many years at Josiah White's when student after student would either be very happy or very sad and angry when their visiting weekend would roll around and their parents did or did not come to campus for a visit. While I understood the feelings of the students then, I am even more attuned to their feelings today because of this experience. Knowing that Kathy was coming gave me something to look forward to and motivated me to care about my future. One thing I can say for sure is that through this experience, having a committed family member there to support me in my care and keep me encouraged along the journey was quite an advantage.

Finally, the big day came. It was January 4, 2021, and I was finally going home. 2020 was over, and 2021 had arrived. I am rarely inclined to wish my life away, but as far as I was concerned, 2020 was a year I was glad to have behind me. Although I learned a number of valuable lessons, there was one in particular that I will mention here. Andy said he was glad to see me angry, because my small, quiet voice from PD was much less prevalent when I was angry. He and others have told me on several occasions that I should get mad more often when I am trying to speak. Even still, it was goodbye and good riddance to 2020.

CHAPTER 8

Flying Solo

I knew I had a long road ahead of me to fully recover. But hey, I was once again a free man. I felt like I had received a get-out-of-jail-free card playing a game of Monopoly!

DeeAnn was staying at our house to help me get settled in our home in Sweetser. She went to work, putting her experience and expertise to good use to schedule in-home health care for me while keeping in mind my PD and its impact on my recuperation. I've learned over the last six years that having Parkinson's factors into virtually every health care decision I make.

As I remember my knee replacement and the importance of going to Washington, D.C., five months later for my Colson Fellows commissioning, this gave me a sense of urgency—a purpose—and a real need to recover my walking ability. I would need that same level of motivation now to regain as much of my old "normal" as possible. But to do this, I needed a great support team, starting with a physical therapist.

DeeAnn called around, trying to find a PT who had specialized training in working with Parkinson's patients. Knowing this would be a long-term partner in my care team, it was important we got this right. She gave me a short list of people to call after a great deal of research on her part. I landed on a young man named Cory Fornal, who is still my physical therapist today, nearly two years after that initial call to him. He has been a genuine gift to me!

Before Andy left, he told me, "Dad, I think you need to write down a little bit of the history of your life prior to all the medical problems beginning in 2017." He thought those who would be working with me should know more of who I was prior to my medical issues. I agreed. So, not wanting to waste any opportunity, I wrote out the same story I've shared with you but included my goals for therapy and desires in finding the right PT and gave it to Cory in February of 2021.

I accomplished three things by writing this out for him:

1. He can see that I am serious about my healthcare.
2. He sees me as a person rather than just another patient.
3. It gave me an opportunity to share my faith.

Since then, I've also given that document to other doctors, nurses, and medical providers. I strongly suggest you do the same.

Adrian "Dee" Gibson Medical History

February 2021

My name is Dee Gibson, and I am a sixty-six-year-old man who has lived a full, good life. I am a committed follower of Jesus Christ and am blessed beyond measure to have three grown children, a committed wife of forty-seven years, and four incredible grandchildren. I was in executive leadership for forty years at Josiah White's, with my last twenty years as the chief executive officer. I retired from Josiah White's in December of 2017. Many of my duties included public speaking and raising money. Over my twenty years as CEO at White's, I managed 300 employees with an annual budget in excess of twenty million dollars. Until I was in my mid-fifties, I participated in three sprint triathlons and lifted weights regularly. Through much of my forties, I played basketball on a weekly basis with a bunch of guys at Josiah White's.

From a health perspective, my life began to change in 2016 when Kathy, my wife, began to notice what I today understand to be bradykinesia and some voice changes (specifically getting quieter). And then in February 2017, life threw me another curve ball when I was diagnosed with thyroid cancer, which resulted in my having two surgeries that ended with having my thyroid removed. Thankful to the Lord, four years later, I am still cancer free. Although I had been under a neurologist's care since early 2016, my symptoms were very mild for Parkinson's disease and no official diagnosis came until the spring of 2019.

In January 2019, I had an elective surgery to have my right knee replaced which was a result of a high school football injury and many years of subsequent use playing basketball with Josiah White's staff and students. While the surgery was deemed a success, still to this day I have some swelling and numbness in my right knee along with my right toes curling down. Depending on what doctor or physical therapist I talk to, it is unclear whether this is PD, knee surgery, or a back-related problem.

In January of 2020, I was playing football with my five-year-old grandson and fell on our driveway. For the next five weeks, I struggled to walk, but the x-rays didn't show any fracture. And then in February of 2020, while turning over in bed, my hip displaced, and I had emergency surgery at St. Vincent Hospital in Indianapolis. Once again, my surgery was successful, but for the next ten months I had four different therapists, each one contributing to my care. I finally felt I was getting back to what was a normal situation for me.

Which brings me to my most recent misfortune. On December 17th, 2020, Kathy and I were T-boned by a pick-up truck who ran a stop sign and hit me square in the driver's side of my car at around fifty-five mph. Having serious injuries, I was sent to Lutheran Hospital in Fort Wayne with a fractured sternum, clavicle, four thoracic vertebrae, numerous ribs, and a large painful bruise on my left leg. After a few days in ICU, I was transferred to Parkview Rehab where I spent the next two weeks in care.

As of this writing, I am now home and preparing to begin outpatient physical therapy. My goals for therapy are that by next October, I hope to be able to walk around my neighborhood (3/4 mile), ride my Trike Bicycle fifteen miles, work out at the YMCA, and get in/out of chairs with ease.

What I am looking for in a PT is:

1. *someone who is committed to helping me achieve these goals.*
2. *someone who is versatile enough in their trade to work on balance/gait issues as well as be able to stretch, do therapeutic massage, and implement Big/Loud strategies as appropriate.*
3. *someone who will become a partner with my neurologist/ortho doctors to help pinpoint what I need to do to help me achieve my goals.*

After spending a week with us, DeeAnn needed to go home and be with her family in Tallahassee. This meant we were going to be flying solo for the first time in nearly a month, and I was glad. It had nothing to do with any of our kids, because frankly I am not sure what we would have done without their help. But DeeAnn's departure represented a return to some sense of normalcy we had not had since the end of November when Andy got married.

Approaching a month after the accident, Kathy and I had both been cleared to drive. And as one might imagine, our driving was close to home and during the daytime hours. We did very little running around, only making trips that were strictly necessary, like doctor's appointments, physical therapist visits, our local pharmacy, and, of course, some of our favorite food hangouts!

As the months passed, I was making good progress, but discovered just how much muscle I had lost and the long road ahead of me. I was going to physical therapy two to three times per week and speech therapy twice per week in the hopes I could meet my goals. I learned during the next six months that regardless of having Parkinson's disease or being in a car accident or anything else, life doesn't come to a screeching halt and wait for us to heal. In fact, Kathy ended up having four surgeries between December 18, 2021 and June 14, 2022, for three separate detached retinas. She was subjected to all kinds of weird sitting and laying down positions for at least a week following each surgery. As it turns out, she will likely have permanent nerve damage in her right eye that will require her to wear a corrective lens. And her eyesight will never be what it was prior to her first detached retina.

Kathy and I had been caring for our aging moms for the previous couple of years. And while most anyone who has had the privilege of caring for a parent in those later years of their life can attest, and as difficult as it is to be responsible for providing the care they need, they wouldn't trade the experience for anything. For me, however, it had another meaning altogether. Being with my mother was like seeing into my own future because she had Parkinson's disease, too.

CHAPTER 9

A Peek of What is to Come?

Although tempting to jump right into the last ten years of my mom's life when I witnessed her living with Parkinson's, it is important that I share with you first about this giant of a person who stood only five foot, two inches tall. I only hope I can live a life that faintly reflects the grace and love she displayed toward other people.

My mom taught me so much about how to handle tragedy with grace and humility. She never lost her zest for life even though she endured many difficult challenges. She was a mother to five children, two of whom she outlived. Her oldest child was a son who had spina bifida. He was always known to me as "baby Gaylin" who died at the age of six months. My mom then had four other children, my three older sisters and me. I was the baby of the family and always considered the spoiled one. Please, don't tell my sisters, but I think they are probably right!

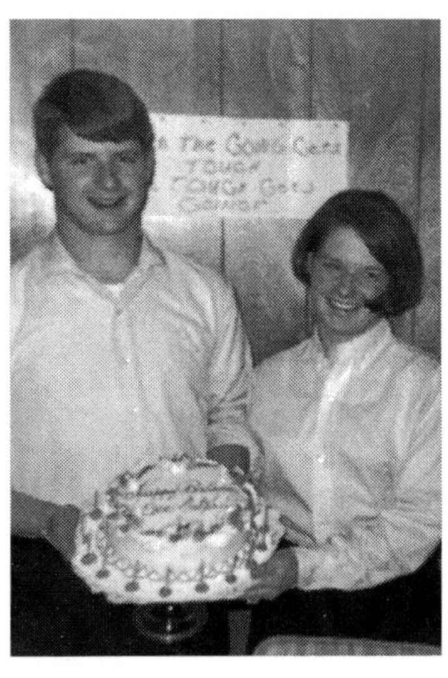

We endured the Palm Sunday tornado of 1965 that completely and utterly destroyed all our family possessions. I was ten years old at the time and have memories of my mom and dad sorting through things in what was left of our family home. When I was twenty-four years old, my next oldest sister died at the young age of twenty-six from a congenital brain aneurysm. She was the mother to two little girls, which was just about as traumatic as it gets.

And yet, even with all of life's tragedies, my mom was able to see the good in life. She was loved by many people. In fact, just recently, a woman I barely knew spoke to me about my mom in the most glowing terms. She may have impacted her friends and acquaintances, but she was most known among her children and grandchildren. Mamaw Gibson, as she was affectionately called by those closest to her, was known for her raucous laughter and her candy cabinet filled with peanut M&M's, Snickers, and potato chips. There is rarely a family gathering where this candy cabinet doesn't enter our conversation. As much as I enjoyed it—and trust me, I did—what I am most thankful for is her gracious and self-sacrificing approach to life.

My beloved mother, who had more than her share of tragedies in her life, had one more hurdle to jump over. She was diagnosed with Parkinson's disease in her late eighties.

While it took a little time to recognize it, it soon became clear that we were dealing with something other than my mom's natural aging process. This began a series of events that transpired over the next seven years, which were some of the most difficult and yet rewarding times of my life. My dad died when he was seventy-eight years old of a heart attack, leaving my mom alone for the next decade and a half. Eventually, my sisters and I encouraged her to move to an assisted living facility because she had begun to fall and was afraid of living by herself. Here, my mom displayed some of the most courageous, gracious, and selfless acts I'd ever witnessed from a person I knew intimately.

Although I'm sure she would have been more comfortable living with one of her children, she made it clear from the very beginning that was not her intention. She said we all had our own lives to live.

At the age of ninety-two, my mother willingly set aside her personal interests by leaving the home she and my dad had lived in for the last twenty-five years, giving up her independence to go into an assisted living facility. This was the first in a series of major life-changing decisions my mom made during the last three years of her life that impacted me greatly.

The second decision came a year later when the facility she lived in determined they could no longer provide the care needed for her to remain there. This resulted in her moving to a second facility that provided more care, but she had to downsize her possessions yet again. Still, she did not grumble or resist her three kids in making this change. I'm confident she knew it was where she would spend the balance of her days on this earth. And then, without warning, my mom was deprived of seeing us because of COVID. We weren't allowed to visit her in person.

She began to fall more often, despite the staff trying to supervise her more closely. With each fall, her paper thin and frail skin would tear, and she ended up with a broken shoulder that never healed. These events took place during the summer and fall of 2020 and the first half of 2021 until her passing.

I was so fortunate to have two sisters who cared for my mom as much as I did. As time wore on, we became more convinced that we needed to find a way for her to have more human interaction. We were done sitting outside of her window, trying to talk on the phone to each other.

After discussions with a resistant administration, we decided to take her out of the home for a day to spend time with us kids. The only repercussion was that mother would have to remain quarantined in her room for fourteen days after returning, which for all practical purposes, she was used to doing anyway. It's a decision we never regretted. And finally, once the COVID scare began to wane, we were able to take mother out of the facility and bring her to our home with no issues. I was so grateful for our transition-free home that allowed her to come and visit us more easily. This was one of the best decisions we made as a family.

I am so thankful I had two sisters to go through this difficult time in our lives. I'm not sure how I would have handled these most challenging times without their leadership and support. My sisters and I are closer today because of my mom's character.

Although not diagnosed until her late 80s with PD, by the end of her life she was displaying many of the symptoms I have today. As I reflect on the last five years of her life, I see a lot of myself in her. I see the problems with her eyes and her quiet voice. I see her inability to navigate through small and tight places and turn around to sit in chairs. Even some of her falls are things I can relate to. Each of these areas grew progressively worse as time wore on. And then this grand woman, who was known for her gregarious laughter and big smile, came to the end of her time on this earth. Even in her dying, my mother was teaching me how to live. She demonstrated a life of abundance, purpose, and meaning not in spite of her circumstances, but because of them.

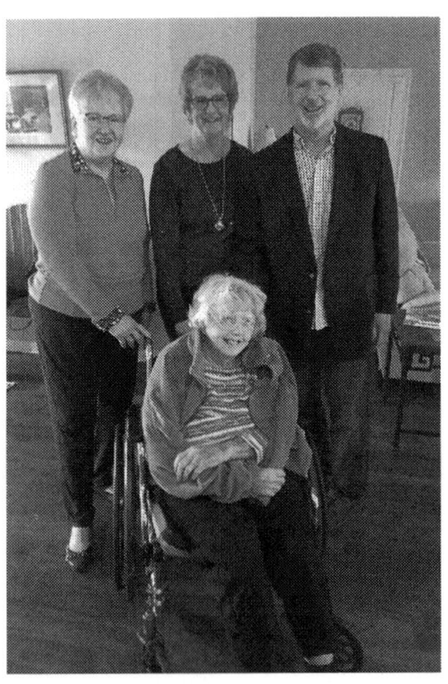

One of the ways I have found my roar in recent years is through my children becoming my voice. In this case, my oldest daughter was able to read the eulogy I wrote for my mother on my behalf.

Mother's Ultimate Gift

As I sat down to write these words, I couldn't help but reflect on my own life as well as Mother's. So as DeeAnn shares these thoughts with you, my prayer is you will receive them as they are intended; as words spoken from me to each of you. Much like it would be if we were sitting down over a cup of coffee, a Coke, or in the case of Gibby and Marshall, apple juice and chocolate milk. I hope you will hear my heart about my mother's ultimate gift.

To some of us she was mother, to others she was mamaw or mamaw-great, to others she was a cousin or good friend . . . to all of us she was adored and loved! Mother gave us many gifts. Some of them were actual gifts, like those gifts back in the late 80s and early 90s when each of us kids got a video camera (and no I don't mean an iPhone) but rather one of those antique kinds that sits on your shoulder and plays a VCR tape. And in more recent years, she would take us kids to Fort Wayne and buy us an "I Love You" gift before taking us out for dinner.

But more important than the material gifts she gave us were gifts that money cannot buy.

The gift of laughter and fun. There were countless card parties with bowls of candy, potato chips, and Coke straight from her candy cabinet. In fact, I wouldn't be surprised if she doesn't have a candy cabinet in heaven just waiting to share it with us someday! Mamaw's laughter could be heard clear across the room or in some cases throughout the theater, like the time papaw flew the paper airplane from the top row of the theater down to the orchestra pit only to have everyone in the 1200 seat theater looking up at us. And of course, we were trying desperately to keep a straight face. Or the time papaw took a picture of his forehead leaving a burn mark. Or even me cuddling up to a mannequin at Von Maur. Mother's laughter was contagious, and she has passed it on to her daughters. Mother's laughter will live on through Penny and Melody for this, I am sure!

The gift of family. Mother loved daddy and all of us kids (that's all of us). I cannot remember a time when she did not put her children before her own needs. Whether it was traipsing through rain, sleet, and snow for all my football and basketball games (from elementary through high school they only missed two games). Or later in life when we would all, and I mean all, pack into that twelve-by-sixty mobile home at the lake. Or even more recently when mother would hold my hand as she lay in her bed at York Place, insisting on a kiss before we left. I knew I was important and mattered to Mother.

The gift of faith and hope. As difficult as life can get and it got pretty difficult for Mother. During her lifetime, she endured great hardship. She lost her first-born son and had a husband who was in and out of the hospital and preceded her in death. She lost all her earthly possessions in the Palm Sunday tornado of 1965. And to the deepest tragedy a parent could ever face as she lost a daughter and two granddaughters. I'll never forget the night Mother called me and said she had some bad news. She had gotten a call from Doug because Kay Kay had died. And how her heart ached for those two little girls who would never have the chance to know their mother. Yet through it all mother never lost hope in her family, hope in life, hope in God.

The ultimate gift was her example of a life well lived as a follower of Jesus. Mother's life demonstrated for us what it means to live a life filled with love, joy, peace, patience, kindness, goodness, faithfulness, gentleness, and self-control. I never doubted Mother's unconditional love for me. Whether it was when she discovered me as a high school kid who was drunk to celebrate my success as being a recipient of the Sagamore of the Wabash Award, I never questioned Mother's love. I always knew she was proud of me and believed in me. And today, as we celebrate her life, I am confident she wants each of us to know that just as she loves unconditionally, so does Jesus. The good news is it's never too late to accept Jesus into our life and we can be the same kind of example as Mother's has been to each of us. In fact, it's not just good news, it's the best news ever!

CHAPTER 10

Cheated But Not Defeated

As glad as I was to say good-bye to 2020, especially since I had spent one month and three days in the hospital during the COVID lockdown, I would be totally remiss if I didn't talk about some of the good things that happened during that year. The biggest event and cause for celebration was our son.

Andy, who was forty years old at the time, came home from traveling the United States on November 10 and informed us that he was getting married two weeks later in our home, the day after Thanksgiving! Andy had finally found his soul mate, the love of his life. Her name is Anja Maree, and she is from South Africa. Our two grandsons affectionately call her "Queen Anja" because of her accent. Andy has known Anja for about ten years, but we didn't get a chance to meet her until March of 2020. Anja came to the U.S. to speak at a Youth With a Mission Conference when COVID hit and was not allowed to travel back to her country for a year. As it turned out, she spent most of that year with Andy and his friends in South Carolina, where he assured us they were just friends. That is, until the first of November, 2020 when he said God told him that Anja was the one girl for him, his helpmate and the one he was to spend the rest of his life with.

While Kathy and I were surprised, we weren't totally shocked either. Little did we know just how important it would be for her to be here, just three weeks after they were married and when we were hit by the truck. Fortunately, we had a good chance to get to know Anja prior to the accident, because afterwards, she became Kathy's primary caregiver while Andy was taking care of me. This is one way to get to know your new mother-in-law! It's not a way I would recommend, but I can tell you it was definitely a good thing for our relationship.

Unfortunately, after our recovery, our time with Andy and Anja was coming to a close. She wanted to travel home to South Africa and share her new husband with her family. So on the fourteenth of February, 2021, after a very hard and tearful goodbye, we put them on a long flight to South Africa, where we knew they would be living for at least two years. In the span of four months, Kathy and I felt like we had gained a daughter and lost a son and daughter-in-law. This was in addition to having just come through a life-threatening car accident. Talk about feeling like Job, an Old Testament Bible character whom God allowed to be tested by Satan. In the course of the book, Job lost his health, his family, and his possessions. Thank goodness, I am not Job!

I was sad that Andy was leaving for at least two years, perhaps more, before I would see him again. Like any good man, I had done a pretty good job of stuffing all those emotions under this tough guy image. But when the day came and I dropped them off at the airport, we stood there with tears streaming down our faces. There were so many things to say, yet not a word was said. And then Kathy and I watched as they walked away with their luggage in tow.

I had so many thoughts running through my mind like a deer scampering through the forest trying to avoid capture. Realizing now more than ever how fragile life is, I wondered if I would ever see him again. What if he got over there and liked it so much he didn't ever come home? Or what if something happened to him while he was there, and I couldn't get there to help like a good father should?

It dawned on me that this is how God must have felt about sending His One and Only Son to this earth for me and you. The difference here is that our heavenly Father knew Jesus' future even before He left heaven and came to earth. I find great comfort in knowing the God who created me understands my pain and suffering in a way that no one else can because He suffered and felt pain, too.

Once I got through the emotional meltdown and regained my equilibrium, I began my recovery in earnest. I had a new goal to motivate me this time. After talking with my two other kids, Andy and Anja invited Kathy and me to visit them in South Africa in the fall of 2021. All three of my kids strongly encouraged us to go. Andy and Anja said if we could get there, they would take care of the rest. So, there it was: I had a new goal. We were going to South Africa in seven months, and I had to be ready to make the trip.

Although I tried as hard as I could during the next seven months, I wasn't able to accomplish all my stated goals before leaving for South Africa. Andy stayed true to his word, though, and made special accommodations for us when we arrived, including a four-wheel scooter for me. Feeling like Mario Andretti at the Indy 500, every place we stayed during our month-long visit had ground floor accommodations or an elevator we could use with the scooter. He also arranged for me to have a massage on three different occasions, which was a highlight of the trip for me. Two of the three massages were at a place called the Botlierskop Game Reserve.

This was unlike any vacation we had ever been on before. It wasn't just a game reserve; it was a resort, and I felt like I was on one of those *Rich and Famous* shows. Kathy and I stayed in a romantic, spacious villa on the game reserve. When we first walked into the room, on our immediate left was a woodburning stove with a fire roaring ever so brightly. Next was a wall of sliding glass doors from floor to ceiling that spanned the entire back side of the villa and led out onto a private deck. And if that wasn't enough, on the other side of the wall was a beautiful tub to soak in while gazing out over the pasture, where you could see the occasional animal grazing on the hillside. The crown jewel of the villa was a private patio with a swing that was also a full-sized bed and an outdoor shower, Kathy's favorite part of the villa. *Ooh la la*, if you know what I mean!! Kathy and I felt as though we had been transported back into the Garden of Eden! PD may take parts of your body, but it certainly doesn't take it all. It certainly doesn't take away your desires, and for that, I am eternally grateful.

While we were on the game reserve, we went on a safari. Our group consisted of roughly twelve people in this big vehicle that was part tank, part Humvee, and part bus. Our tour guide's name was Simba. Initially, I was concerned about how I would get in and out of the vehicle, but that quickly subsided when I realized how helpful the rest of our group members would be when I needed help. While getting into the vehicle, there was a steel ladder you had to climb to get into the seating area. I had to get in and out of the vehicle no less than three times. Each time I felt like a sack of potatoes as they hoisted me up into the vehicle. Andy would help guide my foot up onto the bottom rung of the ladder and then get his arm under my backside and push. Once I got to the top of the ladder, Kathy guided my foot over the railing and one or two of the other gentlemen ushered me safely into the seating area of the Humvee.

Once we were all in the vehicle, we were off into the jungle. The jungle in South Africa might not be what you imagine, with dense trees and foliage—the kind of place you might expect to see Tarzan swinging. Instead, the jungle here is flat, with wide expanses of plains. It's a place where we were truly a part of the animal kingdom rather than man's kingdom. It was everything I had hoped it would be.

We were among some of the most interesting and amazing animals that God created. Simba was very respectful as he drove up to elephants, rhinos, water buffalo, and even a lion. Our group had talked all day about seeing a lion, but Simba held back any guarantees. As the day wore on, we began to lose hope that we might actually get to see the King of the Jungle. But Simba, living up to his name, wouldn't quit until we were able to see this magnificent animal.

As the sun set over the western sky and the cool South African air turned into an almost bone-chilling cold, we finally found one of three lions in the reserve. With dusk approaching, Simba drove the beast of a Humvee faster and faster, which also meant it was louder and louder. The sound of the big diesel engine could be almost deafening at times. That is, until we breached this hill, and there he was—a male lion. Simba throttled down the screaming engine. We sat there for several minutes, watching this magnificent animal. Up until this point in time, the only lions I had ever seen before were in cages at a zoo. This was a totally different experience. In part, because of the respect Simba showed this lion. A big part of the experience for me was being in an open vehicle within twenty feet of this lion. Finally, to complete our day, the lion began to make these huge guttural sounds, not really an all-out roar, but certainly enough to get the idea of what a roar might sound like. It was at this moment I decided what the title of my book would be. After hearing and seeing the majesty of this great animal, I knew that someday I would have a roar of my own.

Kathy and I had talked for a couple of years about going zip-lining at some future date and time. Years before, when we were on another trip and just a matter of hours away from hang gliding off a mountain top in Switzerland, we couldn't go because of some timing issues. Ever since then, we had decided that if we ever had the opportunity, we'd go ziplining together. Well, it was apparent to everyone that I would not be doing that on this trip if for no other reason than we were in a foreign country over 8,000 miles from home. And if something were to happen, that would be bad news. But Kathy was able to go twice, and Andy went once.

I watched my wife on her first ziplining experience. I never realized she was such a thrill seeker until then, but clearly, you don't always know your loved ones quite as well as you think! Actually, it was quite fun to see the smile on her face as she anticipated the trip and even more so to hear her talk of her adventures after she returned.

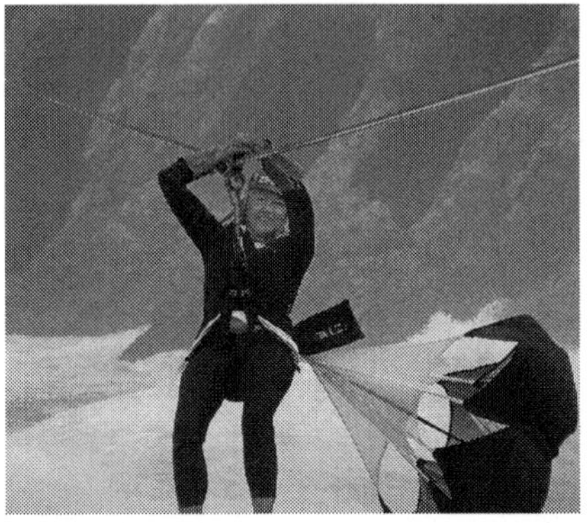

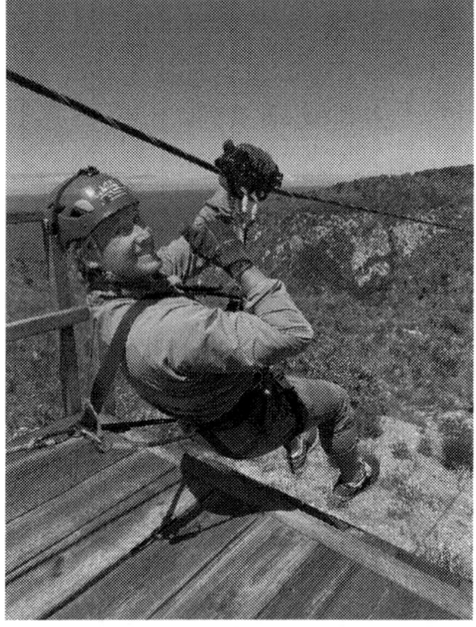

A couple of days later, she went again, but I was unable to watch because the terrain was not handicap accessible. I stayed back at the bed and breakfast, imagining my thrill-seeking wife soaring through the air like an eagle in flight. The videos I watched later were a testimony to this very fact. I also learned that my muscular, six-foot, four-inch, two-hundred-twenty-pound son is not the thrill-seeking, tough guy I had imagined. Rather, he is more of an ostrich—a tough bird who is never inclined to get his feet off the ground!

I was feeling sorry for myself that day, having a pity-party of sorts. Below me was a childcare facility and several different places of business, all busy with the sounds of everyday life. I felt bereft, left behind, and alone while the rest of the world enjoyed their lives. Knowing I needed to process these feelings, I wrote the following poem as I sat in our room:

Cheated But Not Defeated

I've always been taught feelings aren't right or wrong, they just are.
Well, today I'm feeling cheated,
Imprisoned in my perch high above the crowded streets below.

I hear the hustle and bustle of children laughing
And all the locals busy about their day
with not a thought about walking to and fro.

While I am sidelined and all alone, held captive,
My inability to walk has given me cause to feel defeated.

While those I love are off riding a zip line,
I'm resigned to being by myself, killing time.
And while I couldn't be more happy and excited
For my loved ones to have this success,
It is hard to hear their cheer nonetheless.
For the third time this week,
my one and only is doing life without me.

As my thoughts begin to run away

Within the back, dark corners of my mind,
I see a future where the Mrs.
has a life and I'm not in it.

A son who will be relieved when I've gone home,
having a chance to have his independence back.
As more and more of our time on this vacation has past,
I'm feeling as though I'm holding everyone back from having a blast.

But then, I begin to see the reality of this hideous picture in my mind.
It's me not standing up for all that's good and kind.
I have a wife who loves me unconditionally.

A son who has literally held me up
when I could not stand on my own.
I realize there are millions of people in the world
Who have so much less than me.

So what am I to do?
I must count my many blessings,
Name them one by one and resolve anew
Just how determined I must be

To make sure that all those around me
Can see I stand more committed than ever,
to one day again walk with confidence and independence.
Today I may have felt cheated
but certainly not defeated.

The first half of this poem doesn't reflect my feelings today at all, but at the time, these feelings were authentic. I learned many years ago that while your feelings at any one time may seem very real, you can't always assume they are true!

Three weeks into our month-long trip, we received some bad news that put everything into its proper perspective. Kathy's mom, who we had been providing daily assistance to, took a turn for the worse and passed away. Fortunately for us, her two sisters were nearby and took care of all the difficult challenges every adult child faces when caring for the loss of a parent.

We were surprised by her death because she seemed healthy and stable when we left for South Africa. Kathy, her sisters, and her mom even discussed whether she should go, and together, they had decided it would be good for her to take this trip of a lifetime. Although it was a difficult return home with a pending funeral, the time in South Africa and all we saw and experienced there was truly a gift in every way.

CHAPTER 11

A Rocky Road

Several years ago, one of my doctors told me that, having now retired, I needed to make my health my new job. I hadn't realized at the time just how true that statement would become. In the past few years, I have had more than two hundred appointments to see speech therapists, physical therapists, neurologists, orthopedic specialists, endocrinologists, speech doctors, and so on. And this doesn't include my time at the local YMCA. But I had already decided to get the most out of my physical therapy appointments. I needed a reason to go to them. And as it turned out, 2022 would give that to me.

The start of that year was like five of the last six years. It began with yet another hospital stay! I had been seeing my orthopedic doctor regarding pain in my left knee. Ever since the car accident in December 2020, the discomfort had been increasing. So, after much consultation with my care partners (Kathy, my primary care physician, orthopedic doctor, neurologist, and physical therapist), I decided on arthroscopic surgery to repair a torn meniscus. This minor surgery is not a big deal by most people's standards, but when you have PD, no surgery is minor.

My kids gave me a hard time saying that if a football player in the NFL can be back on the field after missing only one game, then surely, I can be ready to at least jog after my surgery. But let's be honest here: I hadn't jogged since before to my thyroid surgery in 2017. And while I had made significant progress over the last year, it was clear there would be no running in my immediate future.

I wanted to make sure I participated successfully in my therapy appointments because Andy and Anja were once again traveling abroad. This time, they asked Kathy and me to join them in Israel for two weeks in October, and how could we say no? We agreed to go as long as Andy promised to meet us at the airport.

With my limitations in speech and mobility, Kathy carried most of the burden of communicating with the airline's personnel and navigating the airport. The upside to needing wheelchair assistance is that we have help from the moment we walk into the airport until we get our bags at our destination.

We landed in Tel Aviv and drove to Jerusalem, where we stayed for the first week. Kathy and I had been to Israel once before in 2007, visiting all the usual tourist sites in Israel. We wanted this trip to be different and were there to spend time with Andy and Anja and experience Jerusalem in a more intimate way. We wanted to soak in some of the culture of the area. After all, these are God's chosen people! And so, we did. We visited the markets, ate the great Mediterranean food, and watched a lot of people.

Once in the old city of Jerusalem, I was issued a motor scooter to make sure we were all able to get around with ease. Riding around on a scooter has pros and cons as not every place is built to accommodate them. But one day at an ice cream shop, this worked in my favor. As we sat outside waiting on our ice cream, we noticed a little boy standing in front of all the many flavors of ice cream saying to his father, "Abba, Abba, can I please, please have some ice cream?" And then it struck me that this is how Jesus of Nazareth likely referred to His Father when He was living back in Bible times (see Romans 8:15). It was a great moment we shared.

Yet another experience we had in Jerusalem was the observance of the Jewish Shabbat. It's the Sabbath, or day of rest, beginning on Friday at sundown and ending on Saturday at sundown. All businesses are closed. Because we were staying in the new part of Jerusalem, we saw firsthand just how busy things can be, and then, all at once, the city became a ghost town. The hundreds of businesses filled with customers became a desolate place within a matter of hours.

On this particular Shabbat, we were fortunate enough to celebrate with an acquaintance of Anja's. Their home was in the heart of the business district, where a throng of people had earlier been busily preparing for this spiritual event in their own homes.

My biggest challenge of the entire evening was ascending to their upstairs apartment. Thankfully, I was able to climb what seemed like a stairway reaching to heaven. It was probably only forty to fifty steps, but they weren't just any steps. They were steep, narrow, and full of twists and turns. Fortunately, I had an entourage of folks assisting me. Kathy and Anja led the way, making sure I was able to navigate the uneven climb, and Andy brought up the rear in case I fell backwards. It was a stark reminder that much of the world is not prepared to assist those of us who are not able-bodied people.

Which leads me to my next big adventure.

One of the reasons we chose to stay in Jerusalem was so we could go into the old city. On the appointed day, we charged the little scooter's battery so we didn't get stranded there. We decided early in our visit to go to the Western Wall, also known as the Wailing Wall, a historic religious site in the city that dates back more than two millennia. It is a place of pilgrimage and prayer for the Jewish people. Many religious and world political leaders have come to pay their respects.

You see, we were walking—well, to be clear, Andy, Anja, and Kathy were walking—and I was cruising along on my scooter. While they huffed and puffed, trying to find their way to the Western Wall, I was in an ignorant state of bliss, merrily along for the ride. Never once did I realize the downward spiral and the obvious necessity of returning to the top of the hill to escape the clutches of the Dung Gate. It is set in the old city's southern wall at the bottom of a very steep hill and provides direct access to the Western Wall. And it was there the following poem was conceived.

Life Can Be Such a Rocky Road

It was a bright and sunny day
As we traveled along our way.
In my four-wheeled chariot
With my son at my side, I was invincible.
Life can be such a Rocky Road.

My little scooter bouncing like a pinball,
Careening over all the bricks.
My emotions tossing me to and fro,
Continuing to wonder, why oh, why
Can't I just get up and walk?
Life can be such a Rocky Road.

Entering in Jaffa's gate,
Imagining how Nehemiah must have felt
trying to understand the hand God's people had been dealt.
All the while wondering what to do,
He prayed and wept asking God to reveal His plan
for him to be an instrument of God's design.
Life can be such a Rocky Road.

Little did I realize on that eventful day,
That going to offer my prayers at the Western Wall
Could be so much like my disease.
Going downhill with ever so little effort
Yet, leaving me with such an uphill climb.
Life can be such a Rocky Road.

But just like Nehemiah, I prayed and wept
trying to understand God's grand design for my life.
Never really feeling like I was heading toward a disaster
Only to wake up to find I was at this bottomless pit
with no way out on my own.
Life can be such a Rocky Road.

But then again, just like Nehemiah,
Whose brother was at his side,
My son came to the rescue
providing a push just at the right time,
propelling me forward and upward toward
to the ground high above the circular road
upon which we traveled.
Life can be a Rocky Road.

Only to be reminded that God's grand design for my life
will only be accomplished with the encouragement and support
of those who know and love me the most.
But then again, life doesn't have to be a Rocky Road.

This story reminds me of Katherine and Jay Wolf's incredibly insightful book, *Suffer Strong*. In it, she writes that we all have wheelchairs. Some of them are visible while others are not. Each and every one of us has someone or something that puts constraints on our lives. For some, it is our marriages; for others, it is having children or not having children; and yet for others, it is our careers. For me, it is PD. The point here is, as was also in my poem, that we were not meant to do life alone. God created us to live in community. And yet, being the self-assured, independent person I am, this isn't something I would have readily learned on my own. We all need others to come alongside to help carry us or give us a boost when we are not capable of doing ourselves. And Parkinson's has taught me that.

The final story to share of our trip to Israel was swimming in the Mediterranean Sea. On the day we went, there were people up and down the beach, just about as far as the eye could see. There were hundreds of lounge chairs with shared umbrellas, and people of all sizes and shapes were ready to soak up some rays. But there weren't any people like me—people unable to walk without assistance.

After a two-mile trek to the beach, we finally arrived. But I could not take my scooter out onto the sand, so I parked it in a small pavilion approximately fifty yards away and shuffled to the umbrella and lounge chairs secured for us. After taking some time to get settled into my new surroundings, Andy suggested we get into the water and swim. I realized these opportunities didn't come up every day, so we meandered our way towards the shoreline. Kathy volunteered to stay with our phones and other personal items.

Once there, I wasn't quite sure what to do with my cane. But not being dissuaded, I promptly threw it to the ground and looked for a familiar arm to grab onto. Andy was right there. He grabbed both of my hands and we proceeded into the water. Walking backward into the sea, Andy held both of my hands until we reached our destination about fifty yards from shore. Once we were there, my son reached up and planted a big kiss on my cheek. I usually wouldn't have thought too much about it, but these weren't normal circumstances. After all, we were on a crowded beach with thousands of people witnessing this entire affair. I've often wondered that if the situation were reversed, would I have had the capacity to show my dad the same kind of affection that Andy showed me.

After about thirty minutes of floating in these sacred waters, we made our way back to shore, where I was able to find my way back to solid ground (if you can call a sandy beach solid ground). Andy, Anja, and I found our way back to our umbrella and chairs, only to find Kathy sound asleep in her chair. I couldn't decide whether to be glad or sad for her apparent lack of concern!

CHAPTER 12

Wise Monkeys

Unfortunately for me, 2022 was not without its difficulties. My symptoms became more pronounced, and PD not only changed the way I viewed my disease but also the way others related to me. One of the biggest challenges during the last couple of years has been my proclivity to fall. Truth be told, I've only actually fallen a half dozen times or so, but if I included my stumbling from a cabinet to the doorway, to a chair . . . then that number would be too many for me to even recall!

Probably the most serious fall I have had since my infamous fall playing football with my grandson in 2020 was when Kathy had gone to Bible study and lunch with a few friends. I was eating leftover Chinese food for lunch and dropped a couple of pieces of rice on the floor. I bent over to pick them up, just like I had done a hundred times before, but this time, I lost my balance and face-planted onto Fred, a Zebra hide whose name was given to him by a good friend of ours. My nose scraped against the fur, tearing the skin, and blood poured out, ruining Fred's beautiful hide. It was not pretty, and I knew Kathy would be home soon. I was bound and determined she would not find me on the floor a bloody mess.

Fortunately, I was able to crawl over to the wooden chair in our foyer and hoist myself up, all the while continuing to drip blood all over Fred and our hardwood floors. I then proceeded to the kitchen, cleaned myself up, and went back to the scene of the crime. I did my best to remain upright as I cleaned the floor, except for Fred, who absorbed my blood and, with every swipe, only spread the stain more widely.

The good news was Kathy came home shortly after I had washed up the best I could. The bad news was I knew I would have to come clean with Kathy and confess to her what had just happened. It didn't take long once she was in the house for her to sense something was out of place. I was just hoping it wasn't my nose!

Within minutes of seeing me up close, she noticed it. And when she saw Fred lying there on the floor with his hide marked with blood, she quipped that she thought Fred had been shot! Kathy went into action and got Fred cleaned up to be as good as new.

Everything returned to normal, meaning my nose healed up. But I felt like something had changed that day. I realized just how quickly things can happen. Fortunately, all I had was a bloody nose and not a broken arm or shoulder. But even to this day, every time Kathy leaves, she tells me to be careful and asks, "Are you good?"

I've often pondered what's behind that question. I think it's because she is always concerned that I might take another nosedive—or worse. She, too, realizes how quickly things can change, and not just for me, but her too! Our lives could come to a screeching halt. More than anyone else, she can see that our hopes and dreams of traveling, going out to eat, and our mobility in general, could be no more. It is sobering to me, too, and frustrating. I can't just get up and walk without worrying her. Or even doing simple things like taking out the trash, carrying a hot cup of coffee to my office, or a myriad of other mundane tasks the average person does without a second thought.

Whether it's walking into a restaurant, a doctor's appointment, or into a friend's home without me using a walker, I realize this has become a major bone of contention between the two of us. She is concerned about me falling, and I just want to have some sense of normalcy in my life without trying to figure out where to park the walker while everyone stares. And to think this is all because I did a faceplant on Fred!

One change that has helped, though, has been a SpeechVive. This is a relatively small device that fits over your ear and looks like a hearing aid or a wireless Airpod. It is designed to help me talk louder by providing background noise when I start to speak. When I first heard about this device, I was somewhat skeptical. But the more I thought about it, the more sense it made.

When you talk to someone who's listening to music, they invariably speak louder when responding to you, and the rationale is the same here. The other reason I was initially hesitant to try SpeechVive is the appearance of it. I had a hard time getting past it looking like an old man's hearing aid. I just didn't want to look like an old man. But what finally convinced me to try it was feeling more and more isolated from people around me because I could not be heard or understood. My results thus far have been mixed. When it works, people tell me they can hear me better, which is great news. But figuring out the technology is another challenge. I've had it for just a short period of time, and it is a learning process of making sure my speech is as clear and distinct as possible so it can pick up my voice. This isn't a cure-all, but I believe it is a step in the right direction. And over time, as I understand what I can do to help make the device more effective, the better off I will be.

I've always prided myself on being a good communicator. In fact, I've been told that back in my prime, when I spoke, it was kind of like when E.F. Hutten did because everyone would get quiet and listen to me. I say this only to suggest I was once a good speaker, and it was an important part of my life and vocation. Whether in small, intimate settings with family or large groups of two hundred or more people for work, I've felt very comfortable sharing complex ideas for the vast majority of my life. All that has now changed. It seems because of my weak and soft voice and the change in my processing and thinking skills, I am quiet most of the time. It's caused me to withdraw from people and conversations.

Another profound impact of PD that even my SpeechVive hasn't been able to fix has been the phone relationship between me and my kids and grandkids. They have a difficult time deciphering what I am saying to them. And given that two of the three kids live such a great distance away, talking with them by phone is the only option. I certainly don't blame my kids, but sometimes I feel left out because when they call home, they always call Kathy rather than me.

It's an even bigger challenge for my grandchildren, especially my two grandsons. They are five and eight, and the fact that they are boys makes communicating with them extremely difficult. I have so many ways I want to speak into their lives, but I just come up short most of the time. Whether telling corny grandpa jokes or trying to corral them when they are with us, I end up conceding all this to Kathy. She is the one they will respond to. But probably the most painful part for me is not being able to talk to them about their values. Kathy is the one who gets to pray with the boys when they stay overnight with us, and I am left out of talking to them about the life changing power of Jesus Christ. This has been a significant challenge for me, but I am so thankful that I am once again finding my roar.

Another recent development has been *blepharospasm*, which causes my eyes close involuntarily. The Cleveland Clinic defines it as "a neurologic disorder affecting the muscles controlling your eyelids. It starts off as twitching and can progress to not being able to open your eyes. Injections help many people get relief."

A year or so ago, I noticed that when I stood in a shower or swimming pool, my eyes would twitch whenever water ran down my face. And when exposed to direct sunlight, my eyes would twitch to the point that my shoulder would shake, causing people to comment on my reaction. Now, my eyes shut involuntarily, and I have to actually use my fingers to pry them open.

Without being too much of a "Debbie Downer" here, there is good news to report on this front. I have had Botox injections in my eyelids. The idea is that the Botox actually relaxes your eyelids making it easier to keep your eyes open. Well, I'm happy to report it has worked wonders for me so far. My understanding is the injections wear off starting around the one-month mark, but I can get these injections on a quarterly basis. This is all very good news for me, because my kids tease me by saying how much younger I look and that I no longer need to use toothpicks to keep my eyes open.

When I tell my story about the quiet voice and sight problems associated with my PD, I often think of the three "wise monkeys" that say, "hear no evil, speak no evil, and see no evil." Well, I've got two of the three completely down and certainly hope I never have the third one.

CHAPTER 13

In Sickness and Health

Where does one begin to talk about the love of their life—especially when it comes to the person who has been not only your best friend, professional sidekick, and lover for the last fifty years but is also now your caregiver and health care advocate?

A while back, Kathy was patiently waiting for me to get out of the car, and she quipped that she had a title for my book: "Life in Slow Motion." We had a good chuckle about it that day and many times since, primarily because this has become an all too familiar theme in our lives in the last few years! What I once was able to do in seconds now takes minutes. And although I've never point blank asked, I'm sure it's one of her biggest frustrations with me having Parkinson's.

I've always been running from one appointment to the next, trying to get one more thing done before my next commitment. After years, no, decades of hurrying from one appointment to the next, now I am perpetually late, which is very frustrating to Kathy. But believe it or not, I really do try to be on time!

This disease has brought home for us both the reality of the sacred lines from our vows, "in sickness and health."

Kathy and I have known each other for most of our lives. We had been friends throughout junior high and high school. In fact, the first time I asked Kathy to marry me was on the steps of a quaint, little country church at my sister's wedding when I was in the eighth grade and she was a ninth grader. And just for the record, she said, "Yes!"

This may sound like love at first sight, but I have to be totally honest with you. Prior to my first proposal to Kathy, I had also thought her younger sister was pretty cute. Being a big country boy, I had a Sears 106cc motorcycle and would drive over to her house and take them both on a ride, sneaking kisses from each of them the whole time! What can I say other than I was a good ole red-blooded teenage boy who tried to make the most of a good thing.

Stolen kisses notwithstanding, some of my best memories of Kathy and me during our younger years were centered around church. I was not very spiritually minded at the time, and Kathy's mini-skirts and great legs kept me coming back to church through most of my high school years.

During the winter of my senior year in high school, God revealed Himself to me, and I knew I had a choice to make. I was two different people: one person to my parents, Kathy, and family, and a different person to my friends at school. The event that led me to really make Jesus the Lord of my life was when I had a good friend over to spend the night. We had become drinking buddies. While my parents were in bed, my good buddy and I were drinking up a storm. In the wee hours of the morning, I told my friend I was going to bed, but I had to go to the bathroom first. The next thing I remember was waking up in the bathtub with my parents standing over me. I had passed out and thrown up all over myself. The only thing I recall my parents saying to me was they would never be able to trust me again. Finally, the double person I was had been exposed, and I knew then I had to make some life decisions about who I was going to become.

I was so embarrassed and ashamed of the person I had become that it took me a couple of years to even begin sharing this life-changing event with anyone else. Today, I tell this story openly and without hesitation because I know this was the beginning of a new life for me—a life that has led to the marriage of my one true love and a career of working with troubled teens.

I am so grateful God used this moment in my life to reveal Himself to me. If there is one thing I am confident of, it's that God can use these painful, intense moments in our lives to get our attention—a topic I'll speak more on in Part III. Suffice it to say, if you have not had a personal encounter with Jesus Christ yet, I really want to encourage you—whether you are twenty-six, fifty-six, or eighty-six—it is never too late to seek the life-changing relationship you can have with Jesus Christ. Having a life with Jesus provides me with a purpose that I would not otherwise have.

So, fifteen months after I made the single biggest decision in my life, I made the second biggest decision in my life. At the ripe old age of nineteen years and three months, while Kathy was a more mature twenty years and six months old, we were going to get hitched, tie the knot, GET MARRIED! I hate to have to admit this, but I really hadn't given our wedding vows much thought. All I knew was I wanted to get married and move on to the honeymoon!

In the years that followed this major life choice, made almost fifty years ago, I have come to think of marriage in terms of four C's: Commitment, Connection, Communication, and Creativity. Jay Wolf writes in his book, *Suffer Strong,* about commitment in marriage, saying:

> "From the start of the idea of marriage, it makes sense to contractually connect two kingdoms or tribes or families through a mutually beneficial agreement when the terms look like these. We will be better, richer, and healthier, and we will love and cherish each other for a lifetime. Yes and yes. Sign here, kiss here. Done and done. But these are only half the story. Whoever wrote the full vows had something entirely different in mind, something far more stunning and valuable than health. To hear a human being covenant to

> another that they will in fact stay even for worse, for poorer, in sickness, until death–should do something to our soul. This is not a contract; this is a commitment that will forever change everything. It's not transactional, it's transformational. (Wolf, 2020, pg. 127-28)"

Jay Wolf goes on to say:

> "Marriage may be the death of me, but it's the birth of we. Maybe it feels like duty sometimes. Maybe it feels like indentured servitude or even prison. Maybe it feels like a ball and chain weighing down every step. And that's why staying when it's hard requires that we make a choice. Not just once but over and over again. But in the choosing and in the staying we will find that what once felt burdensome and confining is actually the avenue to our greatest freedom—freedom from ourselves. (Wolf, 2020, pg. 128-129)"

The second C is *Connection.* Connection is a foundational part of any relationship. It's the building block on which all relationships are built. Having that spark in your marriage is not an option, it's a must! For any marriage to flourish, having the connection that first drew you together must be nurtured and cared for. This is about wanting your mate to know they are loved unconditionally. That your one primary goal is to see them go further and faster in life.

The third C is *Communication.* In order to have any kind of healthy, intimate relationship, with or without PD, you have to have open, honest communication. I have come to believe this is especially true for people who have Parkinson's (or, for that matter, anyone who has a life-changing physical disease or trauma). Honest communication about any number of issues is extremely important. Issues about everything from difficult conversations with doctors to driving to sex, all require good communication skills. And it's more than having the right techniques. As important as they are, it's about having the right attitude, listening for understanding, keeping control of your tongue, and not letting anger rule your mind.

The fourth and final C is *Creativity.* There are many areas where creativity is important in a marriage, but none more so than in the bedroom. Sexual intimacy is an integral part of any marriage.

One of my favorite movies is a 2007 comedy-drama film starring Jack Nicolson and Morgan Freeman called *The Bucket List.* The main plot follows two terminally ill men on their road trip with a wish list of things to do before they "kick the bucket." In this movie, Nicholson has a quote I believe sums up my thoughts on the issue of sexual dysfunction. It goes like this: "Here's something to remember when you're older Thomas; never pass up a bathroom, never waste a hard on, and never trust a fart."

The good Lord spoke of it quite frankly from the beginning of creation when He said that man and woman were to be fruitful and multiply. King Solomon also wrote the book of love poetry called The Song of Songs. Because a person with PD can't move as a person without the disease, whether because of tremors or in my case of muscle rigidity, a person must talk to their partner about what works and what doesn't! This is the most fun part of any intimate relationship. It's about not taking your relationship too seriously. Sexual intimacy is supposed to be enjoyable and fun. As you can imagine, Kathy and I have had some very interesting and fun conversations! The best advice I can give anyone with PD about sexual intimacy is grounded in the four C's: Commitment, Connection, Communication, and Creativity.

Kathy and I have been married just a few months short of a half century. It's amazing to even think of being married for fifty years, but the truth is, it has gone by very, very quickly, especially when I take a few minutes and reflect on our journey. For the overwhelming amount of all those years, Kathy and I worked together, literally side by side. From 1997 through 2017, she was my executive assistant at Josiah White's. She has truly been my helpmate. She not only did all the things one might consider as the traditional role of an executive assistant, but she was also the person I wanted at my side when we were visiting donors, having discussions with board members, and performing many other high-level duties. And most importantly, she is the mother of our three children. She was, and still is, the glue that keeps our family together. In short, I married up when I married Kathy. And even now, after almost fifty years, she is my helpmate today more than ever.

At no time in our first forty-five years of marriage did I ever consider there would be days she would have to help me put on socks because I'd be too stiff to bend over and get my socks over those size thirteen feet of mine. Lest anyone get the impression that our marriage is perfect, I can tell you it is not. After all, we all live on this side of heaven and at times we can all be selfish, spiteful, and prideful. But any of these things that come up from time to time are quite small in comparison to the good we see in each other.

I often get asked to share the key to a great marriage. And more often than not, I say, "My job is to help her go further and faster in life." In other words, it's my responsibility to put her hopes and dreams ahead of mine. And the second is to not major in the minors. I have found there are very few things in life worth fighting over.

I think it is appropriate here to quote some of the key verses in the love chapter of scripture. 1 Corinthians 13:4-7 says:

> "Love is patient and kind. Love is not jealous or boastful or proud or rude. It does not demand its own way. It is not irritable, and it keeps no record of being wronged. It does not rejoice about injustice but rejoices whenever the truth wins out. Love never gives up, never loses faith, is always hopeful, and endures through every circumstance. (NLT)"

I only hope I can model these verses as well as my one true love has. One thing I can say with confidence is that my capacity to receive this kind of love is greater because I have PD. You see when I no longer have my independence, it is then that I am most capable of receiving this kind of love. And for that, I *will be* eternally grateful!

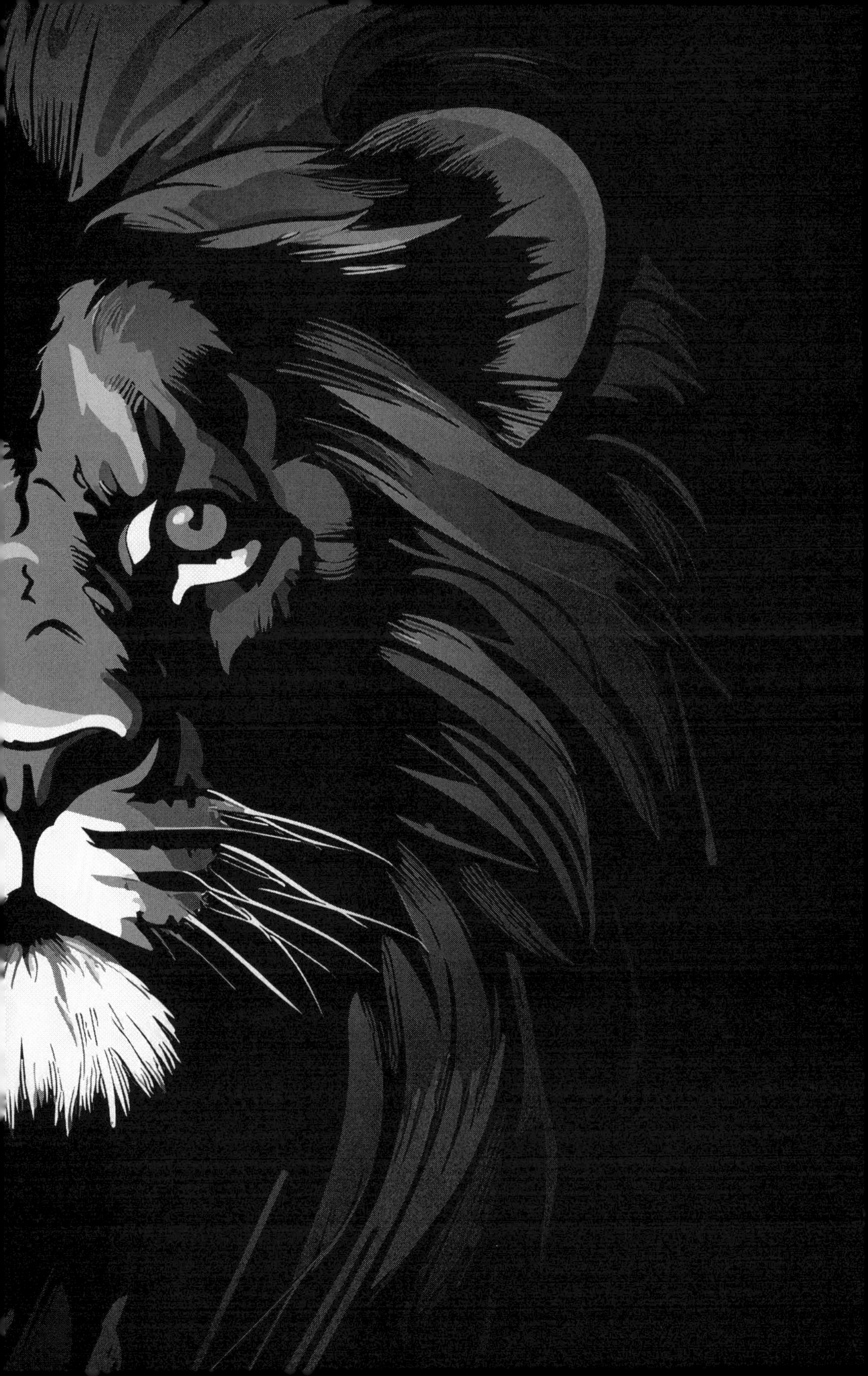

PART 2

Life in Slow Motion

CHAPTER 14

Kathy's Story: In Her Words

Where does one begin to write about how this disease has affected us? When you watch the love of your life struggle with basic physical tasks, like putting on shoes, a sports coat, and so on, you learn that each day is a gift, and you can choose how you will respond to it.

Our lives have slowed way down. I remember one time when we were getting ready to leave for church, Dee was in his office working on his computer. As I would normally do, I gave him a ten-minute warning, then a five-minute warning before it was time to leave. When it was time to go, I went into his office and said, "Come on, hon, it's time to leave," only to have him say he still needed to brush his teeth. After doing so, we proceeded to the car, and he opened the car door and just stood there, frozen. After a couple of minutes, he slid into the car, and we finally were off to church. Ten minutes late to church, again!

When you find yourself in this or a similar situation, what steps can you take to navigate the endless doctor appointments and therapies just to keep what mobility you have from getting worse? Let me share with you eight ideas that have helped us immensely.

1. **Keep a robust, but realistic schedule:** We have continued physical therapy, voice therapy, and massage. Use everything at your disposal to help minimize symptoms. In planning our days, we try to only do one or two things that require going

somewhere, mainly because by late afternoon whatever energy we had is fading. So, we are careful not to schedule too much.

2. **Keep going:** Early in Dee's diagnosis, his symptoms were mild, and life was pretty normal overall. We just continued to do our regular schedule with extra exercise to prolong the mild symptoms as long as we could. However, in early 2020 when Dee fell and broke his hip, then in December of 2020 when we had an auto accident, his condition escalated, and it was hard to get back what he lost during that time. Through it all, Dee has never wavered in his persistent attitude of "never give up." Even though it takes him a long time to do basic tasks, he still does them.
3. **Keep control of what you can do:** Honestly, I don't baby him, and I try really hard to be his helpmate and not his caretaker. I encourage Dee to speak for himself as much as he can even with the softness of his voice and the speed of his talking. I am not quick to step in and translate. While he has been passionate about writing this book, it has been a bit of a struggle for me because I am a very private person. But I am incredibly proud of all Dee has accomplished.
4. **Keep laughing:** We laugh a lot because sometimes struggling with the simplest things is funny. So don't take these moments too seriously. For some reason, when I help Dee put on his compression socks in the morning, this daily ritual has become funny. So, we begin our day laughing. It hasn't, however, always been this way. In the beginning, I was frustrated that I had to help, and I just wanted him to be able to do it himself. I thought he should just try harder. At some point, I realized it wasn't his fault. Now, he is still able to put them on; it is just faster if I help!
5. **Keep doing normal things:** We traveled to South Africa in 2021 and Israel in 2022. Crazy . . . right? We have wonderful memories and no regrets. We enlisted help from family to make it happen, so don't be afraid to ask for help. We are so thankful for our family,

who drops everything to help when we need it. If you don't have family readily available, reach out to trusted friends.

6. **Keep exercising:** Why is this so hard? This has proven to be very helpful. So, get up and do something. Take a walk or a bike ride. In the summer of 2021, we got Dee an incumbent bike with pedal assist. This has been so good for both of us! Make plans to get outside and enjoy nature because moving has been beneficial for everyone's health.

7. **Keep leaning into your faith:** Our faith in Jesus has carried us through and gives us hope to face another day. We don't have to stay worried or sad. Instead, we can choose today to live our lives with joy and peace, knowing the God of the universe loves us! Some days are easy, and sometimes we fail, but making a moment-by-moment decision to trust in the One who gave His life for us makes all the difference.

8. **Keep being grateful:** Gratitude changes a person's perspective. Because no matter how bad it is, you can find something to be grateful for. I have written down what I am thankful for from time to time, and it really is helpful. I'm thankful that over the last few years, Dee has always been kind, loving, and never complaining. He just perseveres each day, and it truly has been a labor of love to go with him on this journey. We don't know what the future holds, but we are in this together. Our *life in slow motion* isn't so bad. We have everything we need and more. Our retirement years are not what we planned for, but we have learned to adapt our expectations and wait and see what the Lord is planning next.

When my kids were very young—probably eight, five, and three, I had a Superman beach towel. It traveled with us wherever we went on vacation: to Niagara Falls, to Florida, and certainly to Lake Webster. My kids thought I could do no wrong, and I took full advantage of the opportunity, convincing them I was Superman, but only during the night when they were asleep.

Obviously, I told them I couldn't use my real name without drawing too much attention to myself during the daytime, so I used my fake name of Dee Gibson *rather than* Clark Kent. *I even had them convinced that I could run faster than a speeding bullet, fly, and even jump over tall buildings in a single bound. The only thing bigger than my imagination was my capacity to tell all these little white lies to my young, vulnerable, naive, and impressionable children! It took only a matter of a few weeks, however, for my three kids to discover that their dad had been "pulling their leg" the entire time.*

CHAPTER 15

DeeAnn's Story: Superman's Kryptonite

He was Superman. Growing up at Josiah White's, with dad holding various leadership roles, he always told me he was really Clark Kent and under his button-down dress shirt was the proof. When getting ready to leave to attend to a crisis or swim in the on-campus pool, he'd say he had to go—he was Superman. And to me, he was. Dad has always been a big, strong man.

A star high school football player for the Marion Giants, Dad always looked the part—even after having kids and working his nine-to-five (or supposed nine-to-five). He always lifted weights or played basketball with the kids and staff on campus, and we all enjoyed our time at the pool. He continued to be Superman with his voice, standing up for at-risk youth across the state of Indiana for forty years.

I'll never forget that one day he mentioned to me that these kids can't vote, and someone needs to be their voice. I'd never thought about it that way. Politicians receive zero votes or dollars dealing with at-risk youth, and Superman was saving them the best way he knew how. He served and advocated for them with politicians, in courtrooms, and with donors.

The first signs that something was not right started in about 2012-2013, or maybe even a bit before. It turns out our Superman had kryptonite. The first thing I noticed was a decrease in facial expressions. I remember telling my husband, "Dad just needs to quit that job. He's so unhappy all the time and that stress is going to kill him. It's really taking a toll. He never smiles and laughs anymore."

In hindsight, those were likely early signs of his disease. It was easy to write it off as stress, anxiety, and depression, as he had many strenuous events during that time as the CEO at White's. The state government was significantly changing the pay structure for care, and staff layoffs weren't out of the question. Looking back, I think those were likely the early signs something was wrong.

When I think of Dad before Parkinson's, I think of him as active, talkative, and quick to smile and laugh. I mostly think of him as Superman, a CEO speaking, running meetings, and operating a large non-profit. I think of him tubing with my girls at the lake, swimming and driving the boat, wearing his Superman cape. I think of long conversations over things that matter.

My family and I moved to Florida in 2012, and I remember either the first or second fall after we moved, Mom and Dad came for a visit. My husband, Brady, and I were shocked and concerned with what we noticed. Dad was very slow to eat and cut his food, and he struggled with fastening his seat belt. He would get the seat belt so close to the buckle and just sit there. The alarm would start dinging and we'd think, "Just buckle the seatbelt!"

He also just seemed to walk more slowly as well. Dad has always been late to things, so it wasn't totally abnormal, but we noticed a difference. After they left, Brady and I discussed whether to say something to them and if so, what. I decided to call them once they arrived back home, and they reluctantly admitted that Dad was having some issues. They were doing some tests for more information. But while Dad was still CEO at White's and knowing they were extremely private, they kept most everything to themselves. They often didn't share things with us kids, and they certainly didn't share it with anyone else.

For a very long time, Mom and Dad denied anything was wrong. Yes, he was having symptoms, but they were not typical of Parkinson's, and Dad didn't have a diagnosis. As time went on, though, he began struggling more and more to express himself with his voice. Those around him at work began to notice and suspect something was not right. Eventually, Dad started making his exit plan from White's—much sooner than he had planned. This kryptonite was really doing a number on him. He was going to retire.

Retirement has not been what he and Mom planned. However, I do think they've made the best of it! Dad has continued to decline physically with each major surgery and a car accident, which has hastened difficulties. He just can never get fully rehabilitated. At some point, they seemed to accept the Parkinson's diagnosis, and Dad started taking medication he said didn't help. His voice has continued to get worse, and he has been more difficult to understand.

This is one of the biggest ways his diagnosis has affected me personally. We've been robbed of meaningful communication, those discussions over the things that matter and those that are just part of the everyday. His difficulty with speaking and expressing himself makes it more challenging for us. I don't live close by, and I can't just stop in to talk with him, sitting close and studying his lips when he's speaking. Our conversations primarily happen via text or phone, and neither of those are very conducive to his struggles. FaceTime helps, but even that is difficult some days. Our conversations have gotten less and less frequent. We rely on Mom, who is hard of hearing but refuses to get hearing aids. Yes, they are quite a married pair. He can't speak very well or loudly, and she can't hear!

This has changed our relationship for sure; for the most part, I don't think for the better. I miss the old conversations. He is so wise and has so much to offer with his perspective. I'm so thankful for our ability to email and text, as this has been what we've had to do, though I'm still sad about it. As my girls have gotten older, there have been times I've called to talk about how to handle a situation, and he's listened and said he'd send me an email. That works, and I'm thankful for that, but I do wish we could just have an easy conversation like we used to.

I know Dad prays for us, and even if he can't talk to us very well, the Lord knows what he is saying and hears his prayers. This may be the most significant way he can be involved in our lives right now.

I would be lying if I said I don't ever question why my Dad has this struggle, but mostly, I've just accepted that because we're living in a fallen world where there is sin and death, there are diseases and trials of all sorts. This is just the one our family is dealing with. I pray for a miracle, and then I pray that if it's not God's will for us to have a miracle on this side of heaven, God would give us all the strength, wisdom, and grace we need to endure this trial. I pray that we glorify God in it and that He would use it for His glory and to point others to Him.

I think I already wrestled with these issues a lot when my mother-in-law passed away due to cancer. I've come to terms with the fact there is pain and suffering in this life, but we have hope this isn't all there is! We have a hope and a future in Jesus Christ. As believers, we will live forever in a place with no suffering, no pain, and no tears when Christ returns. We will have a new heaven and a new earth, and all will be made right. I have hope that Jesus loved us so much, He died so we might live, and He conquered all sin and death. This is just temporary. I still wish my dad didn't have to suffer from an illness like this and that my family didn't have to watch him lose his ability to walk and talk. However, I have confidence that He reigns and will be with us in these trying days and the ones that lie ahead.

CHAPTER 16

Andy's Story: The Gentle Giant

I remember being a little boy and having this one mental picture of my dad while I was growing up. It was a beautiful summer day, and we gathered by the lake for vacation. My dad always took a Superman beach towel with him, playfully convincing us kids that he was indeed Superman. I had my doubts, but one day, standing on the boat dock, I watched as my dad sped by in a vibrant yellow Rinker speed boat, the Superman beach towel tied around his neck like a cape, fluttering in the wind. At that moment, I was convinced he was, indeed, Superman.

While you have had the opportunity to read about his imposing physical presence and how Parkinson's has taken it or the way he used to be able to command a room, he was unquestionably a remarkable man; there are so many things about my father that people didn't see! As a kid, I vividly recall him vacuuming the carpet on many Saturday mornings and assigning us kids to dust the living room, understanding that our mom wanted it done. Most mornings, I would walk out of my bedroom to get ready for school, and he would be sitting on the back porch or in his favorite recliner with his Bible on his lap. He never missed a ball game and would drive my little sister one hour each way to volleyball practice multiple times per week. He was fiercely protective, gave us room to fail, and extended grace when we made mistakes. He loved us kids immensely as we grew up and continued to support us through college and into adulthood, being the perfect sounding board as we got older.

While this was never the plan, I took on the role of assisting them in their travels. If not for Parkinson's, I might not have had the opportunity to travel the world with my parents. We were lucky enough to hear a lion roar, watch dolphins play, float in the Dead Sea, lounge on the beach in Tel Aviv, and witness him ride a camel overlooking the Dome of the Rock, thinking he might fall off the entire time. I'm the one with amusing anecdotes about pushing my dad up a very steep hill because the electric scooter didn't have enough power and joking that he needed to lose some weight. Or, one of my favorites is the time my wife, Anja, saw way too much of my father's business because he didn't fully shut the bathroom door and was too slow in pulling his shorts up as she walked in on him. All he managed was a quiet "Sorry about that!" and a belly laugh!

People don't see the awe and wonder in which they live now even being dealt these circumstances in their lives. Traveling has been these big flashy moments where nothing seems impossible, but it's in the mundane moments when their true character shows. For instance, Dad has always been known for being late. You are getting ready for church, and everybody is heading for the car, and then suddenly, Dad has to brush his teeth, and now we are all late! Well, now it is even worse. He still thinks he is faster than he really is. I watch my mom pull out a stopwatch and start timing how long it takes Dad to get in the car to see if he can beat his last time. Go Superman!

You hear them laugh all the time. You will hear them in their bedroom laughing, and you know that something ridiculous just happened. The way they still love and serve each other is something truly remarkable.

It is an honor to be their son, and even up until this day, they are still Superman and Lois Lane to me.

CHAPTER 17

Denae's Story: The Lifelong Leader

So here we are—my turn to write a chapter of this book. Honestly, I didn't want to write it. In some ways, I have put it off because of family obligations and the intensity of my husband's and my careers. But I know myself, and if I was honest, I understand writing it down forces me to think, feel, and deal with the realities of my dad having Parkinson's.

Of course, my family has technically been dealing with his diagnosis for years. Each of us has had our part in supporting and participating in the various stages, complications, and daily hurdles. But for me, this experience is different from my other siblings. I am the kid who lives full-time near my parents and worked side-by-side with my parents for over a decade. I am the kid who has slowly watched this disease take over his body and dramatically change my parents' lives. I often think of this process as watching someone lose small amounts of weight over time. You almost don't recognize the changes because they are slow, consistent, and over time. But I see the disease progression daily. The reality or complexity of dealing with Dad's Parkinson's hasn't been something I just have to sit down to think about. Well, that was until now.

So, where do I begin? My siblings shared stories about Dad being Superman. Those are core memories of Dad for all of us kids. My specific memory was the Superman beach towel he always used at the lake, telling me it was a part of his cover story. But I will fast forward to sharing a different version of Superman: Dee Gibson, the executive leader. I had the privilege of working with my dad for over ten years. He was one of the typical movie-type executives who usually wore a suit and tie. He was the kind of leader summoned to Indianapolis to use his voice at the state house, advocating at the legislative level for work. Then, run back from Indianapolis to campus or one of the satellite offices to facilitate a meeting. To close work, just in time to head to town to hold a church board meeting. With the day finally ending, he would head home to help mom, take me or a sibling to a sport's practice, or get a workout in before bedtime. In all aspects of life, Dee Gibson was a leader. His character was evident everywhere, and whether at work, church, home, or in his marriage, Dee Gibson showed up the same: steady, caring, and capable.

Sure, over the years, my dad's diagnosis changed our relationship. If there was one thing Dad and I could always do, it was talk, and I mean talk. Whether we were in meetings, planning, strategizing, or hanging out, we could always find something to discuss. Dad is a ferocious reader and learner, regularly forwarding us kids or just me a recent article he read about leadership. Or send us all a podcast from one of his favorite authors with a new insight into faith and culture. Dad is one of those people everyone reaches out to for advice or to get his insights on a situation. He can see things from many different perspectives and help guide you to the next steps. Dad used his voice to advocate for kids and families in crisis at the highest level. He used his voice to share knowledge of leadership and business operations. He ran an organization for over forty years, inspiring many to give their time, talent, and financial resources to a Christ-centered mission. Again, he used his voice to share his love and radical belief in Jesus Christ as he went about his everyday life. Dee Gibson spent most of his time using his voice for the good of others.

Over the years, Parkinson's has dramatically affected his ability to speak, write, and read to some extent. One of the things I miss the most is hearing my dad speak. What I would give to be able to call and chat about all things nonprofit and social sector business or to have an in-depth conversation about a hot topic, social issue, and the intersection of faith like we had in the days before Parkinson's. As much as I miss those conversations, I want you all to know I have come to learn and love the value of his presence. Although the relationship has changed in so many ways, and we both have learned to grieve the loss of the days when conversations were easy, there is something to be said about him just being in the room, on the call, or sitting in the chair listening to you. Although the disease has taken a lot from him, his character has remained: steady, caring, and capable. And, when you are with him, you feel seen, loved, and cared for.

While I could probably write a whole book about the journey our family has been on through my dad's Parkinson's diagnosis, the request was only to write a chapter. We have all learned a lot over the years. Unfortunately, the learning has come at his expense. So, instead of writing a whole book, I will give you all the Cliffs Notes and a version of the lessons I have learned through this process.

Lesson #1: Don't wait until you retire. We all "know" in our minds that we shouldn't put off the dream trip, taking more time off to see friends or family is important, and we shouldn't wait to learn a new hobby or chase after that dream. There is a big difference between "knowing" or "experiencing" it. I realize that I am not the one with the illness, so technically, I have no idea what it would be like. Still, I have watched my parent's retirement look very different from what anyone would have wanted or guessed. If anything, I will be way more proactive and intentional with this next phase of my life. I know my parents have no regrets about their life before Parkinson's, but this has been a constant reminder not to wait until I retire because I might not get the retirement I want or hope for.

Lesson #2: Character matters, and we find out who has it during suffering. I have watched my parents embrace this difficult journey with love, faith, and perseverance. Their character hasn't wavered. Losing yourself could be challenging when times are hard and the future is unknown. I often wonder, "If I got diagnosed with a life-altering disease, would I still be able to choose joy? Would my faith remain as strong?" I had many questions about how I would show up if this were me. I sure do hope and pray that if, by some chance, this was how my life would go, I would show up like my parents.

Lesson #3: Love and marriage get tested when "shit" gets real. Many say wedding vows like, or in the spirit of, "for better or worse, in sickness and in health, til death do us part." And the longer you are married, the more real those vows become. My parent's love story is one for the movies. I always knew their marriage and relationship were special; however, watching them through this process has only reminded me of their deep love and what it takes to live out that life in real time, regardless of the circumstances.

Lesson #4: Grief can happen slowly and silently. A lot of times, we think of grief when something traumatic happens or when problems or issues arise for some time. But I never really thought about how grief can happen slowly and silently. This is my experience. My dad's Parkinson's has gotten worse over time, and I have been around them a lot during all of it. I never fully realized the grief that comes with it. There are so many times I grieve the fact that my kids never got to experience, or really won't remember, Dad not being sick. Other times, it hits me when I'm on a call or trying to have a discussion, and I just miss the ease of how it used to be. But it isn't like this traumatic event; it is just the silence and slowness of it that hits and wakes up all the buried feelings of disbelief, anger, sadness, and acceptance of reality.

Lesson #5: Own your health and health care. Watching my parents navigate a very complex, time-consuming, and messy healthcare system is something else. Learning to advocate for quality care and owning the right to determine your own health and medical intervention is critical.

Lesson #6: Have an appreciation for the community of people, the resources, and access to care. Having a support system and people you can count on is one of the Lord's most precious gifts. My parent's siblings all live close by and have participated in so many ways throughout this journey. Over the years, they have crafted a beautiful community of lifelong friends, former co-workers, and a church family who continue to care, support, and pray for our family. Often, with my job, I see the effects of living in the United States without resources, whether tied to access to healthcare or doctors, transportation, or finances. There have been so many times I have found myself in awe of how blessed we are to have the ability to travel to doctor's appointments and pay for technology or equipment that enhances our lives.

Lesson #7: Your siblings can save you. I can't fathom this journey with my parents without my brother and sister. They say your siblings are your best friends for life, which is true for us. Whether it is calls, webinars, research assignments, hospital stays, or support over the years, my siblings, who live in other states or even countries, are always there. I may be the one living the closest and the first responder, but I am far from doing this alone.

Lesson #8: Faith remains. I am not sure why our family's journey had to include Parkinson's. I am not sure we will ever know the reason. So often, people wonder why bad things happen to good people. Or they question God's sovereignty. Or question His nature of love during difficult times. Honestly, I don't have the answer to many of those questions. All I know is what I have experienced and seen, and I have seen a God show up in how my dad lives his daily life with Parkinson's. I have seen my mom love and care for my dad with love that transcends reason other than her faith. I have experienced my brother and sister drop everything and come home to help. I guess I am saying I have seen Jesus being lived out. Having faith isn't about having all the answers or having no doubt. Having faith is believing when you don't have all the answers and have all the reasons to doubt. Faith ultimately boils down to trust. It is trusting that Jesus Christ is who He says He is, regardless of our circumstances and the limitations of our own ability.

So, for the Gibson family, faith has, faith is, and faith will remain as we navigate each step of this journey.

To sum it all up, one of my dad's favorite Bible verses, Joshua 1:9, states, "Have I not commanded you? Be strong and courageous. Do not be afraid; do not be discouraged, for the Lord will be with you wherever you go." The Lord never promises that life will be easy, but he does promise to be with you. I pray my family can be strong. I pray my family can be courageous. I pray my family will live and not be afraid. I pray my family will honor, but not dwell, in discouragement. I pray the Lord our God continues to be with us everywhere we go.

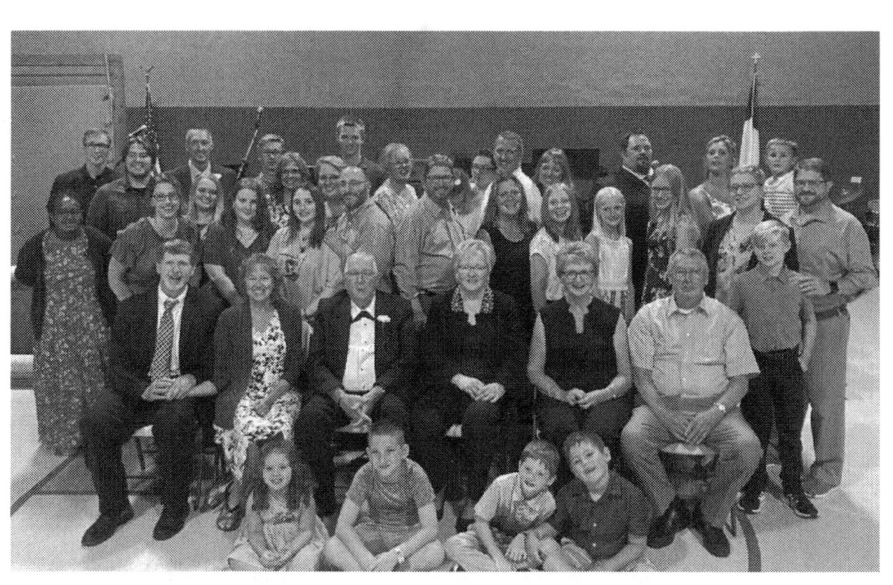

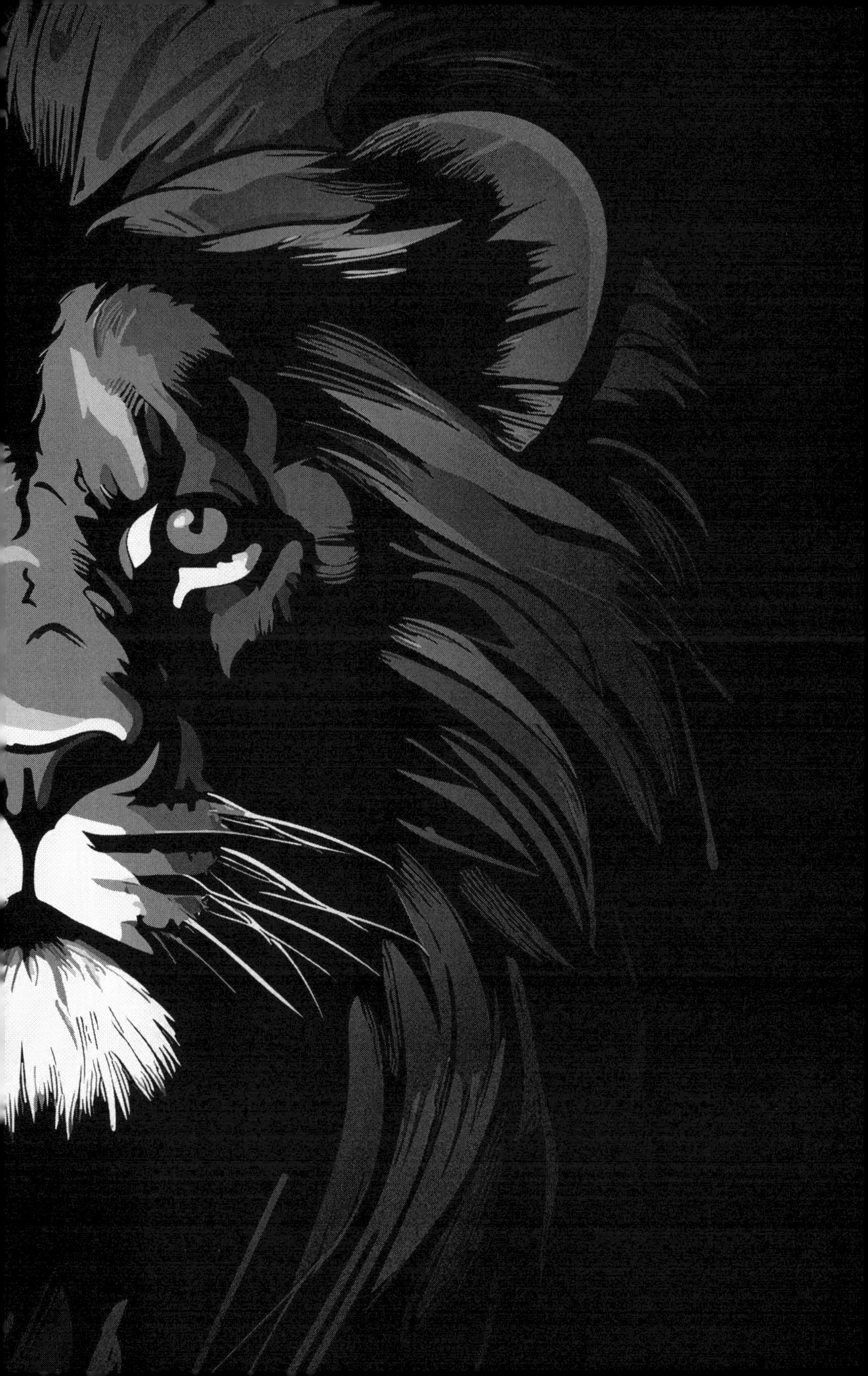

PART 3

Is There Purpose in Your Pain?

CHAPTER 18

Worldview Matters

My mom had entered hospice care sometime before her actual passing, but they promised to keep her comfortable. She had already decided not to have any life-sustaining measures. I'm grateful because by the time she entered care, she could no longer make those decisions for herself. And for any of you who have gone through this with your parents, you know exactly what I am talking about!

It was extremely difficult watching the woman who brought me into this world slip into life everlasting for what seemed like an eternity. I wrote in my journal that, for the first time, I was watching life slowly leave a person and was devastated at how terrible death can be. I remember thinking there has to be more to life after death. It can't mean that's the end, right? And I'm sure many of you are wondering where this is all going. You thought this was a book about PD . . . and it is! But in reality, it is about much more. It's about life, both now and in eternity!

Parkinson's has forced me to slow down long enough to contemplate what I believe and why I believe it. You can't adequately address the full implications of this diagnosis without talking about the grief and loss that goes with it. You lose your physical abilities, your independence, and your future hopes and dreams.

The significance of having the freedom to grieve your losses cannot be overstated. In his insightful little book, *Good Grief,* Granger

Westberg identifies ten steps in the grief process. For the purposes of this book, I am going to focus on four of the steps.

The first step is being in a state of shock or denial, thinking, "This could not be happening to me." The second step is depression, which is anger turned inward. The third step is anger turned outward, where our emotions finally surface, and we show anger toward others who have accepted our loss and moved on with their life. And the last step is affirming reality. Westberg goes on to say that anyone who goes through significant grief comes out of it a different person.

As difficult as it is to adapt to the physical limitations of PD, it is less of a challenge than dealing with the emotional, mental, and spiritual side. I believe a person can come to terms with their disease, and eventually, their physical handicap becomes a new normal. However, talking about the emotional and spiritual side can be more difficult, primarily because you cannot see, touch, or feel it.

Since my retirement, my mom's passing, and my health challenges, I've questioned if there is any purpose in my pain. But to answer the question, I've had to ask some foundational questions. Is there a God? Does He care about me? Does He know about me personally or did He create us to fend for ourselves? Or is there no God at all? Are we simply a blob of cells, randomly created by no one or nothing?

The late Charles "Chuck" Colson, a hero of mine, is the founder of the Colson Center for Christian Worldview. In his book entitled *How Now Shall We Live*, he suggests the world can best be described as having a four-part story: Creation, Fall, Redemption, and Restoration. According to Colson, these categories cover the central questions that any worldview must answer:

Creation: Where did we come from, and who are we?

Fall: What has gone wrong with the world?

Redemption and Restoration: What can we do to fix it? (Colson, 2004, pg. xiii)

Colson contends that the Christian faith is the only faith big enough to handle life's big questions. A significant number of people have asked me questions. Do you ever wonder why God let this happen to you? Why do you think God allows bad things to happen to good people? Or they say things like, "Dee, you don't deserve this." Quite frankly, I needed to be able to answer some of these challenging questions for myself as well as for others. Colson adds:

> "As agents of God's common grace, we are called to help contain and renew his creation, to uphold the created institutions and society, to pursue science and scholarship, to create works of art and beauty, and **to heal and help those suffering from the results of the Fall.** (Colson, 2004, pg. xii, emphasis added)"

I have buried myself in reading or talking to those afflicted by PD, or some type of debilitating disease, in an effort to answer these pesky questions, hoping my disease may be of some benefit to you.

I am of the conviction that what we believe about the purpose of pain in our lives has as much to do with our worldview as anything. When I was in college some fifty years ago, I took a philosophy class. While the professor didn't use the word "worldview" per se, he posed three questions that I recognize as foundational for all of life and constitute our worldview. They are: Where did I come from? Why am I here? And where am I going? Whatever perspective we take to answer these three questions determines how we believe the world works.

To help better understand how worldview impacts our daily lives, I'd like to go back to my days in residential treatment with teens in crisis. At Josiah White's, the youth in the program had endured traumatic life events and many faced drug abuse, poor school performance, depression, suicidal ideation, gang violence, and physical and sexual abuse. The result was a skewed worldview. It left them believing their life script had already been written, ensuring they were destined to return to the dysfunction their parents or community had given them.

This view of life was very powerful for them, yet it was not accurate. Nevertheless, it often dominated their lives.

A second influence that caused me to consider if there is any productive reason for this pain was Michael J. Fox's book, *No Time Like the Future: An Optimist Considers Mortality.* Actually, it's what inspired me to write this book.

The public nature of his bout with PD, and his work with the MJF Foundation, encouraged me and thousands of others in the same battle. For the last three years, I have been a regular listener to the Foundation's webinars that air every third Thursday of the month and are very helpful and informative. Although I doubt we have much in common in the area of politics or faith, I still feel a kindred spirit with him because we share the journey of Parkinson's disease! We also both have an incredible family, spent time in Africa, lost a close parent figure, and have had a host of other health problems. All these things happened in what he called his "annus horribilis," or year of disaster or misfortune, causing him to question his trademark optimism for the last three decades. He said, "Over the coming months, I will feel a shift in my worldview, and struggle to believe in the ideas that I've espoused for years. My optimism is suddenly finite" (Fox, 2020, pg. 159-160).

Michael shares a few stories and then says, "I'm beginning to see that faith, or fear's opposite, can be expressed as gratitude, which has always been the bedrock of my optimism" (pg. 200).

This is the first place where we disagree. I have really struggled to understand what he means when he says the opposite of fear is faith and that faith can be expressed as gratitude. It seems to me the only way a person can repel fear is with love—the love of the One who created us. When talking about mortality, the only faith that really counts is faith in the Author of life, the Source of our lives.

Then Michael's view of mortality comes full circle. He is standing in front of a huge crowd of people at the MJF Foundation Gala. Fox writes:

> "I'm looking out at the sea of faces again. It strikes me that whenever I'm beating myself up over a personal setback, or feeling ineffective in my life, I need to reflect on this moment—this panoramic view in front of me—which is the result of an instinct to help, to embrace a community, and to try to make a difference. Good things can come from bad things (pg. 219-220)."

In this, I can agree with Michael wholeheartedly. He then wraps up his book with final thoughts on mortality:

> "When I visit the past now, it is for wisdom and experience, not for regret or shame. I don't attempt to erase it, only to accept it. Whatever my physical circumstances are today, I will deal with them and remain present. If I fall, I will rise up. As for the future, I haven't been there yet. I only know that I have one. Until I don't. The last thing we run out of is the future (pg. 226)."

This is the second time I find myself in disagreement with Michael, and where I feel our worldviews are literally worlds apart. When he writes that he knows he has a future until he doesn't, it's troubling. This may be a great turn of phrase, but nothing could be more serious than to address one's eternity. This nonchalant comment seems so out of place for the weightiness of the conversation.

At the same time, I really do value Michael's obvious love and great relationship with his wife and kids. I also admire his perseverance and sense of gratitude toward life and all that comes with walking out Parkinson's each day.

These last few sentences are where I want to leave my thoughts on Michael's book because I do respect and appreciate his heart for those struggling with PD.

> "Really, it comes down to gratitude. I am grateful for all of it—every bad break, every wrong turn, and the unexpected losses—because they're real. It puts into sharp relief the joy,

> the accomplishments, the overwhelming love of my family. I can be both a realist and an optimist (pg. 226)."

In my journey over the past two years with this disease, and since beginning the writing of this book, I have wrestled mightily with the question of pain and suffering. And my goal in this final chapter is to bring it all home together and answer some of those pesky questions about the purpose of pain in our lives.

CHAPTER 19

Loved

A number of years ago, when I worked in residential treatment, we had a program for teenage girls called Compass Rose Academy. It was an incredible program, and we would periodically host weekend retreats for them and their parents. During one of these weekends, each girl had a clay pot in a cloth bag, and they were instructed to break it with a hammer. Once the clay pot was broken, the girls were asked to put it back together using gold-colored glue. The purpose of this exercise in the Japanese art of *kintsugi* was to help them see that they can take those shattered pieces of their lives—lives broken by shame, false guilt, peer relationships, and abuse—and put them back together again to create something more beautiful than the original. They were reassured that they don't have to be perfect to be loved.

Hopefully that message is equally clear to those of us who have PD. I believe God can take the broken pieces of our disease and make us into someone who is more life-giving and brilliant than we were prior to it. We just have to be willing.

In his excellent essay featured in *Plough Quarterly* titled "God's Purpose in Your Pain," Pastor Rick Warren reflects on his son who tragically took his own life. Warren suggests that when confronted with some kind of pain or suffering, people typically have one of two reactions: they either run toward God or away from Him.

Before we go any further, let's address two fundamental questions. You may be wondering if there is a God and if so, does He know who you are.

I am convinced there is a God who loves me and knows me by name. Allow me to share four reasons that I know this to be true:

1. **Recognizing creation.** All nature cries out that we are a created people. Everything from a beautiful sunset to a majestic mountain range to the complexity of our own body points to a creator, God.
2. **My own life.** I can see the change in my life over the years, leading me to becoming a better man.
3. **Intense research and reflection.** I've given my worldview a great deal of thought, studied the works of many people, and have come to the conclusion that there is a God.
4. **Faith in God's Word.** I believe the Bible to be true and that it can be trusted to inform our lives on what is reality.

You will notice that reasons one and two are more experiential in nature and what I personally believe to be correct, while reasons three and four are more intellectual and academic in nature. My faith is grounded in a solid foundation. It can address all of life's biggest and most difficult questions, all the while recognizing it is still a matter of faith.

For anyone interested in knowing more or going deeper into my journey, I have included a listing of resources at the end of the book for your further exploration. There, you will find a list of authors, philosophers, and apologists that I have studied. There's also a list of scriptures I have found to be true and helpful in knowing the reality of Jesus, including His death on the cross and resurrection three days later.

So, why does God allow bad things to happen to good people? First, my experience is that pain and suffering are common to everyone. When I was the director of Josiah White's, I used to tell people that we all know someone who is struggling with some kind of abuse, emotional distress, or mental illness. Whether sharing with a large group or individuals, there was universal agreement. I believe the same is true with people who have PD or any other type of debilitating disease. The reality is that suffering is part and parcel of the human experience.

Second, suffering is the great equalizer of all humanity. Every one of us is battling some kind of pain or suffering, although I find that most Christians struggle to admit this. So often, it seems they pretend to live a perfect life in front of other people, hiding their problems and covering up their sins. The result is they are viewed as being hypocritical and fake. Everyone already knows we don't have it all together.

> "We can choose whether we will waste our pain or learn from it and use it to help others. Instead of asking yourself, "Why is this happening to me?" start asking God two other questions: "What do you want me to learn?" and "Whom do you want me to help?" (Warren, 2023)."

We get to choose how we will respond to God's plan for our lives. As for me, I am choosing to believe in His goodness and that great things are in store for me and my family.

Wintley Phipps is an incredible vocalist, and he sings some great traditional Christian hymns. One of my favorites is his rendition of "It Is Well With My Soul." During one of his performances, he told the story of a flight attendant he met and her hardship. And he shared this incredible quote that speaks to me in a very personal way. He said:

> "It is in the quiet crucible of your personal, private sufferings that your noblest dreams are born, and God's greatest gifts are given in compensation for what you've been through (Phipps, 2012)."

My prayer for you today is that you will seek out the only One who can answer life's deepest and most profound questions you are struggling with today. For it is when we find Him, we find comfort in the journey. And knowing I am loved by my family and in a right relationship with God . . . I firmly believe that everything is going to be alright.

EPILOGUE

A Life Worth Living

As Kathy, my kids, and grandkids have walked with me through the journey of writing this book, there have been many family meetings, tears shed, and lots of laughter. The good, the bad, and yes, even the trials I have suffered along the way, will be a testament to the goodness of the God who sustains all of life.

I pray for my children and grandchildren, that they will not live in fear of an uncertain future because they know Who holds the future. And He is a good God! My hope and prayer for each of them, and you as well, is that in some small way, your lives will be brighter and filled with the unspeakable joy that can only come with a relationship with the Author of life.

ACKNOWLEDGMENTS

My caregiver team includes my wife, three adult children, grandchildren, sisters and their husbands, sisters-in-law, and two nephews. As I stated in the opening of my book, the closer you are to living with someone who has PD, the more your life will be impacted.

Thus far, you have heard me talk about Kathy, my better half for the last fifty years, and read her words regarding this unexpected journey. You have also heard, in their own words, directly from my three adult children. I appreciate them sharing from the heart.

I am very fortunate to have two older sisters, Melody and Penny, who live in the area with their respective husbands, Lee and Ronnie, both who have been more like brothers to me than your typical in-laws. Each have been married for over fifty years. My sisters bore the brunt of taking care of my mom. In addition, Melody has been my chauffeur, taking me to the doctor, the airport, and various therapy appointments when Kathy could not. I've very grateful for these four.

Melody also has two sons, Kevin and Kraig. Kevin has been such a big help to me over the last several years. Up until two years ago, he would use his four-wheel drive pickup truck to take my boat to the lake. But more importantly, Kevin makes me feel like I am important to him. He could see my health was failing, so he anticipated my needs and volunteered to help me when he knew I could offer him nothing in return. Well, except a little bit of "quiet fellowship" where, between us, we put away a pizza big enough for a family of five. Kraig is a ministry leader and allows me to feel like I can still contribute to his life by sharing my experiences in fundraising, personnel, and board governance. Thank you, boys.

Jim Spangler and Jeff Schumacher are two of my very closest friends who have been there for me, prayed for me, and accepted my lack of contributions to most every event we've been to together in the last couple of years. I first met Jim fifty years ago. We had just graduated high school and met while working at the Grant County Highway Department. We became fast friends during that first summer before going to college, and he and his wife, Darlene, are still very close personal friends. One of Jim's greatest strengths is his loyalty. For instance, I sent him the following text message and his response reveals his faithfulness to our friendship.

The text reads as follows:

> *Dee: Hey Jim, you've been on my mind ever since we were together a couple of weeks ago. You are such a great friend. Everything from helping me get into the car, to not being able to hear me, to me having my eyes close involuntarily. I'm sure it's got to be hard and frustrating for you. I know it is for me. Thank you for being such a good friend.* 🙏😊
>
> *Jim: You are very welcome. Nothing has changed since we first became friends. Friends are when you enjoy doing things with and being around each other. The other things can and have been accepted and disregarded as life, but to me not detrimental in the least to our friendship and never will. Merry Christmas, my friend.*

This exchange exemplifies the kind of friendship Jim and I have with each other. Since this text now many months ago, Jim has continued to demonstrate his commitment to me as a friend. He makes coping with this dreaded disease just a little bit easier!

Jeff Schumacher is a second, very close friend I've known for twenty years. We initially became professional friends as we both served on a national board of directors while CEOs of nonprofit agencies working with children and families in Indiana. Over the ensuing years, our wives became close friends as well. Jeff and Tina introduced Kathy and me to the art of drinking wine, be it ever so rarely! Over the last five years, as my disease has progressed, our friendship has only deepened. He is an excellent listener and a man of deep faith, which means the world to me. As we were getting ready to leave a get-together at their home, Jeff called us all to the center of their living room, and we had a time of prayer where he specifically prayed for me and Kathy. And when he recently learned that I was going to see another neurologist for a second opinion, he sent me the following text:

> *Dee, I understand you will be going to Cleveland clinic tomorrow. I will be praying for clear minds for the doctors and a clear path forward for you and Kathy. Love you brother!*

I'm guessing for both Jim and Jeff, those text messages (and more importantly, the heart behind them) weren't any big deal. But I can tell you as the one on the receiving end of those messages, they meant the world to me. Thank you, friends.

And then there are the Three Amigos from Josiah White's. Each of these men have had an incredible impact on my life. They are three of my most trusted friends with whom I had the privilege of working.

Byron Brunn was Josiah White's CFO. He and I would spend hours together after work, commiserating about the ministry and its future funding. Terry Hyden was the director of technology. He is a self-taught IT guy who knows more about putting networks together than anyone I have ever known. And Tony Brown who was the director of support services. He is one of those guys who knows a lot about everything to do with building maintenance. But for me, they are more than just friends I worked with. These are truly my spiritual brothers, and I can look forward to seeing them in heaven. These three were some of the first at Josiah White's with whom I took the risk of sharing my health struggles. They each extended their sincere concern to me, and I never worried about them keeping my condition confidential.

To anyone starting their journey with PD, I'm sure you recognize the importance of having people in your life who you can trust with something as personal as actually uttering those dreadful words, "I have Parkinson's disease."

And then finally, there is Jay Driskill. Jay and I worked together for more than thirty years. He was the vice president of residential services and lived on our campus as my next-door neighbor for most of those years. Jay probably doesn't realize it, but he was my mentor, particularly from one perspective. He is one of the most disciplined people I know with his own level of fitness. He was super dedicated to his eating habits and physical training. Although not a big guy, Jay was also one of the strongest people I've ever known (kind of like Arnold Schwarzenegger). Jay would encourage me to get out of my office and into the gym or weight room. Occasionally, he would shame me into it, but most of the time, he was a great encouragement and very inspirational. To this day, he still is. Whenever I see him, which is never often enough, he always shows genuine concern and offers to pray for me.

There is also a whole host of people who I have never met before, but have been so gracious to me at restaurants and in other public spaces: giving me extra space, opening doors for me, and offering assistance when I am struggling.

And finally, no discussion of my care team would be complete without sharing with you who they are. Care partners are those professional individuals who have/are contributing to my life in a professional capacity.

First on the list is my primary care physician, Dr. Jim Orrell. He has known me for many years, and I now consider him a friend as well as my primary physician. I see Dr. Orrell at least two times per year, and he never fails to provide both excellent care as well as encouragement. He has such a positive attitude about getting me the care I need and providing spiritual encouragement. On a recent visit, Kathy and I mentioned the difficulties we were having with getting a script for a motorized scooter. He immediately wrote us one and then shared what an encouragement I had been to many people. I had no idea.

Cory Fornal is my physical therapist. Of all the ones I've had, he is the best. What I appreciate most about Cory is his capacity to not give deference to my PD over my back and hip problems. He is quite capable of handling whatever conditions I present. He never deals with the impact of one without considering the complicating factor of the other. I also really appreciate his positive attitude. Cory has a light-heartedness in his approach to my treatment that fills me with optimism and hope I've not seen in others.

My speech therapist, Ms. Leslie Butterbaugh, is also an incredible pathologist. She mixes the right amount of push with the right amount of understanding. I've long since passed the point of feeling embarrassed about yelling in her office while others there are probably wondering what in the world is going on. Leslie gives me exercises to do, which I confess are rather boring and I sometimes skip them, but I understand the importance of consistently making this effort.

And last but not least are my neurologists. Over the past several years, I have gone to the I.U. Med Center which is a teaching hospital. Most of my care has been delivered by resident doctors who are supervised by more tenured neurologists. The ones I've seen are there for a couple of years and then move on either to another rotation or graduate and go into private practice. In the early stages of my disease, this was fine. But in the last couple of years, as I have needed more specialized care, I am currently transitioning to another neurologist who will hopefully provide me with greater consistency.

It has often been said that it takes a village to raise a child. Well, it also takes a village to care for someone who has a debilitating disease like PD. And I feel very fortunate to have this group of people in *my* village.

RESOURCES

WHAT IS PARKINSON'S DISEASE?

According to the National Institute of Health and Institute of Neurological Disorders and Stroke, Parkinson's disease (PD) is a movement disorder of the nervous system that gets worse over time. As nerve cells (neurons) in parts of the brain weaken, are damaged, or die, people may begin to notice problems with movement, tremors, stiffness in the limbs or the trunk of the body, or impaired balance. As symptoms progress, people may have difficulty walking, talking, or completing other simple tasks. Not everyone with one or more of these symptoms has PD, as the symptoms appear in other diseases as well.

There is no cure for PD, but research is ongoing, and medications or surgery can often provide substantial improvement with motor symptoms.

WHAT ARE THE SYMPTOMS?

The four primary symptoms of PD are:

1. Tremor—A tremor (or shaking) often begins in a hand, although sometimes a foot or the jaw is affected first. The tremor associated with PD has a characteristic rhythmic back-and-forth motion that may involve the thumb and forefinger and appear as a "pill rolling." It is most obvious when the hand is at rest or when a person is under stress. This tremor usually disappears during sleep or improves with a purposeful, intended movement.

2. Rigidity—Rigidity (or muscle stiffness), or a resistance to movement, affects most people with PD. The muscles remain constantly tense and contracted so that the person aches or feels

stiff. The rigidity becomes obvious when another person tries to move the individual's arm, which will move only in short, jerky movements known as "cogwheel" rigidity.

3. Bradykinesia—This is a slowing down of spontaneous and automatic movement that can be particularly frustrating because it may make simple tasks difficult. Activities once performed quickly and easily—such as washing or dressing—may take much longer. There is often a decrease in facial expressions (also known as "masked face").
4. Postural instability—Impaired balance and changes in posture can increase the risk of falls.

PD does not affect everyone the same way. The rate of progression and the symptoms differ among individuals and typically begin on one side of the body. However, the disease eventually affects both sides, although symptoms are often less severe on one side than on the other.

People with PD often develop a so-called parkinsonian gait that includes a tendency to lean forward, taking small, quick steps as if hurrying (called festination), and reduced swinging in one or both arms.

They may have trouble initiating movement (start hesitation), and they may stop suddenly as they walk (freeze).

WHO HAS PARKINSON'S? (STATS FROM PARKINSON.ORG)

- Nearly one million people in the U.S. are living with Parkinson's disease.
- This number is expected to rise to 1.2 million by 2030.
- Parkinson's is the second most common neurodegenerative disease after Alzheimer's disease.

- Nearly 90,000 people in the U.S. are diagnosed with PD each year.
- More than ten million people worldwide are living with PD.
- The incidence of Parkinson's disease increases with age, but an estimated 4% of people with PD are diagnosed before age fifty.
- Men are 1.5 times more likely to have Parkinson's disease than women.

ONLINE RESOURCES

- Parkinson's Disease Caregiver Information: https://myparkinsons.org
- The Michael J. Fox Foundation for Parkinson's Research: https://michaeljfox.org
- Parkinson's Foundation: https://parkinson.org
- American Parkinson Disease Association: https://apdaparkinson.org
- Cleveland Clinic: https://clevelandclinic.org
- Speech aid for people with PD: https://speechvive.com
- Northwest Parkinson's Foundation Speak Up app: https://nwpf.org/resources/speak-up-app
- Speech, physical and occupational therapies for Parkinson's disease: https://lsvtglobal.com
- Training for people with Parkinson's disease to use their body more normally: https://rocksteadyboxing.org
- Tips For Improving Communication in People with Parkinson's Disease: https://my.clevelandclinic.org/health/articles/9392-speech-therapy-for-parkinsons-disease

WRITTEN RESOURCES

- *Walking with God through Pain and Suffering* by Timothy Keller
- *Suffer Strong* by Katherine and Jay Wolf
- *How Now Shall We Live?* by Charles Colson and Nancy Pearcey
- *God Grief* by Granger E. Westberg
- *Overcoming Adversity* by Joni Eareckson Tada
- *The Dopamine Journals* by Dr. John P. Williams Jr.
- *No Time Like the Future* by Michael J. Fox

HELPFUL SCRIPTURES

- 2 Corinthians 12:7-10 (TPT)
- James 1:2-4 (TPT)
- Romans 8:18 (TPT)
- John 9:1-3 (TPT)
- 1 Peter 4:12 (TPT)
- Psalms of Lament (Psalm 6, 10, 12, 13, 22, 38, 42, 43, 86, 130)
- Job 1-42 (NLT)

ENDNOTES

Cleveland Clinic. N.D. "Blepharospasm." https://my.clevelandclinic.org/health/diseases/21546-blepharospasm. Last updated May 21, 2021.

Wolf, Katherine and Jay. *Suffer Strong: How to Survive Anything by Redefining Everything.* Grand Rapids, MI: Zondervan, 2020, 127–129.

Colson, Charles. *How Now Shall We Live?* Carol Stream, IL: Tyndale House Publishers, 2004, xii–xiii.

Fox, Michael J. *No Time Like the Future, An Optimist Considers Mortality.* New York, NY: Flatiron Books, 2020, 159–226.

Warren, Rick. "God's Purpose in Your Pain." *Plough.* https://www.plough.com/en/topics/faith/discipleship/gods-purpose-in-your-pain. Last updated March 2, 2023.

Phipps, Wintley. "It Is Well With My Soul." April 6, 2012. https://youtu.be/E8HffdyLd0c?si=NYwNYAs9k8rmNly6.

National Institute of Neurological Disorders and Stroke. N.D. "Parkinson's Disease." https://www.ninds.nih.gov/health-information/disorders/parkinsons-disease#:~:text=Parkinson's%20disease%20(PD)%20is%20movement,the%20body%2C%20or%20impaired%20balance. Last updated January 8, 2024.

ABOUT THE AUTHOR

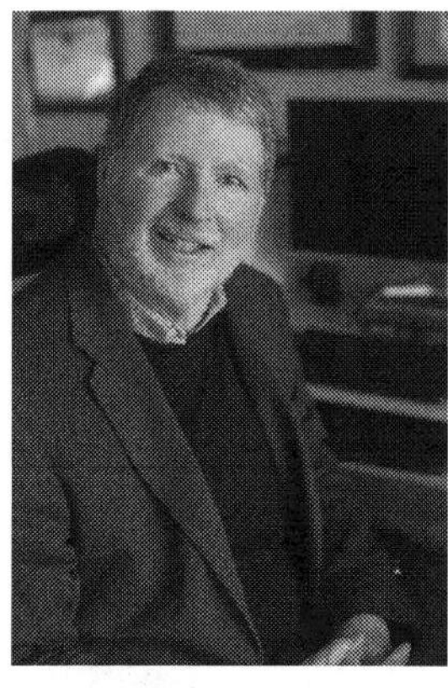

Dee Gibson has dedicated his life to serving others for forty years, twenty of those as chief executive officer at Josiah White's, a 170-year-old organization and one of Indiana's oldest and largest nonprofit social services agencies. He has served on numerous boards and committees dedicated to the welfare of children including the 2004 Indiana Commission for Abused and Neglected Children and their Families. Dee finished his remarkable career receiving one of Indiana's most distinguished awards, The Governor's Sagamore of the Wabash, recognizing individuals who make significant contributions to their communities and whose qualities and actions endear them in the hearts and minds of Hoosiers.

Dee is a graduate of Marion College (now known as Indiana Wesleyan University) in Marion, Indiana, and has a graduate degree from Ball State University in Muncie, Indiana. He is a licensed social worker in Indiana as well. In 2019, Dee was commissioned as a Colson Fellow, from the Colson Center for a Christian Worldview. This is a ten-month deep dive into culture and how it relates to a Christian worldview that provides Colson Fellows with clarity, confidence, and courage to effectively engage the world.

Although Dee struggled with symptoms of Parkinson's disease for several years prior, he was not formally diagnosed until 2019. Since then, he has suffered numerous setbacks. But with the incredible support of his wife and children, he has continued to make "lemonade out of lemons."

Dee and Kathy Gibson have been married for fifty years. They have raised three children, DeeAnn Hanlon, Andy Gibson, and Denae Green, and share four grandchildren together. Today, they reside in Sweetser, Indiana, and continue to live a vibrant life dedicated to their families and serving others. They attribute their lives, legacy, and journey through Parkinson's to their relationship and faith in Jesus Christ.

Made in the USA
Middletown, DE
22 November 2024